AF811985

# Dhat Syndrome

Sujita Kumar Kar • S. M. Yasir Arafat
Vikas Menon
Editors

# Dhat Syndrome

## Medical, Psychological and Sociocultural Aspects

Springer

*Editors*
Sujita Kumar Kar
Department of Psychiatry
King George's Medical University
Lucknow, Uttar Pradesh, India

S. M. Yasir Arafat
Department of Psychiatry
Enam Medical College and Hospital
Dhaka, Bangladesh

Vikas Menon
Department of Psychiatry
Jawaharlal Institute of Postgraduate Medical
Education and Research (JIPMER)
Puducherry, Tamil Nadu, India

ISBN 978-981-99-8869-3 ISBN 978-981-99-8870-9 (eBook)
https://doi.org/10.1007/978-981-99-8870-9

© The Editor(s) (if applicable) and The Author(s), under exclusive license to Springer Nature Singapore Pte Ltd. 2024
This work is subject to copyright. All rights are solely and exclusively licensed by the Publisher, whether the whole or part of the material is concerned, specifically the rights of translation, reprinting, reuse of illustrations, recitation, broadcasting, reproduction on microfilms or in any other physical way, and transmission or information storage and retrieval, electronic adaptation, computer software, or by similar or dissimilar methodology now known or hereafter developed.
The use of general descriptive names, registered names, trademarks, service marks, etc. in this publication does not imply, even in the absence of a specific statement, that such names are exempt from the relevant protective laws and regulations and therefore free for general use.
The publisher, the authors, and the editors are safe to assume that the advice and information in this book are believed to be true and accurate at the date of publication. Neither the publisher nor the authors or the editors give a warranty, expressed or implied, with respect to the material contained herein or for any errors or omissions that may have been made. The publisher remains neutral with regard to jurisdictional claims in published maps and institutional affiliations.

This Springer imprint is published by the registered company Springer Nature Singapore Pte Ltd.
The registered company address is: 152 Beach Road, #21-01/04 Gateway East, Singapore 189721, Singapore

Paper in this product is recyclable.

# Preface

Dhat syndrome is known as a culture-bound syndrome identified in South Asia. People with Dhat syndrome often present with anxiety and distress related to semen loss. This is often accompanied by multiple somatic and sexual symptoms. The symptoms of Dhat syndrome have close resemblance with other neurotic and stress-related disorders. Myths related to sexuality are often the core phenomenon in Dhat syndrome which is responsible for the psychopathology. Addressing the myths mostly results in the resolution of the syndrome. However, many patients require pharmacological and psycho-social management. Due to strong cultural beliefs and myths associated, often patients with dhat syndrome reach to traditional healers, before getting the proper psychiatric consultation, resulting in further consolidation of their myths and poor attitude towards treatment. Although dhat syndrome resembles a male entity, a similar entity has been also reported in females, where females attribute their non-pathological vaginal discharge to psychological distress. The pattern of symptoms has a significant resemblance with dhat syndrome in males. The syndrome has been affecting not only sexual life but also the overall quality of life, especially in South Asian culture. However, there is no standard book that exclusively discusses various aspects of the syndrome, indicating an academic under-prioritization. We aimed to discuss all the possible aspects of Dhat syndrome. Hence, this book fills the gap as well as it is a unique and useful book for this syndrome. It discusses the evolution of the concept of Dhat syndrome to current understanding and its management.

We start the book with the phenomenological aspects of the syndrome. Subsequently, we discuss the epidemiology, nosological contradictions, how Dhat syndrome evolves in the Indian subcontinent, course and outcome, comorbidities, help-seeking behavior, conditions mimicking dhat syndrome, assessment, pharmacological and psychosocial management, Dhat syndrome in females, public health aspects, current research status, and controversies highlighting whether it is a myth. We tried to prepare stand-alone chapters as well as to maintain links among the chapters. For that, there might have been some overlaps of content even though we were careful about it.

This book will be useful for readers of allied disciplines who are interested in cross-cultural psychiatry (e.g., psychiatry, psychology, sexology, dermatology, urology, gynecology, adolescence health, mental health nursing, anthropology, philosophy, social sciences, epidemiologists, and public health professionals). Postgraduate students, doctoral students, and postdoctoral researchers from other disciplinary fields will also find great value in this work.

Lucknow, Uttar Pradesh, India Sujia Kumar Kar
Dhaka, Bangladesh S. M. Yasir Arafat
Puducherry, Tamil Nadu, India Vikas Menon

# Contents

1 **The Phenomenology of Dhat Syndrome** . . . . . . . . . . . . . . . . . . . . . . . . 1
Ravi Philip Rajkumar

2 **Epidemiology of Dhat Syndrome** . . . . . . . . . . . . . . . . . . . . . . . . . . . . . . 19
Swapnajeet Sahoo and Rahul Chakravarty

3 **Dhat Syndrome as a Diagnostic Category: The Nosological Struggle** 29
Sujita Kumar Kar, Vikas Menon, and S. M. Yasir Arafat

4 **Dhat Syndrome in Indian Traditional Medicine** . . . . . . . . . . . . . . . . . 37
Deblina Roy and Shubha Joshi

5 **Course and Outcome of Dhat Syndrome** . . . . . . . . . . . . . . . . . . . . . . . 49
Surendra Singh Rajpurohit and Naresh Nebhinani

6 **Comorbidities Associated with Dhat Syndrome** . . . . . . . . . . . . . . . . . . 61
Adarsh Tripathi and Saumya Upadhyay

7 **Care-Seeking, Pathway to Care and Disease Burden in Dhat Syndrome** . . . . . . . . . . . . . . . . . . . . . . . . . . . . . . . . . . . . . . . . . . . . . 73
Amit Singh

8 **Assessment of Dhat Syndrome: Clinical to Behavioral** . . . . . . . . . . . . 85
Sandeep Grover

9 **Entities that Mimic Dhat Syndrome** . . . . . . . . . . . . . . . . . . . . . . . . . . 95
Yukino N. Strong

10 **Pharmacological Management of Dhat Syndrome** . . . . . . . . . . . . . . . 105
M. S. Bhatia and Aparna Goyal

11 **Psychosocial Management of Dhat Syndrome** . . . . . . . . . . . . . . . . . . 115
Om Prakash and Shipra Singh

12 **Female Dhat Syndrome** . . . . . . . . . . . . . . . . . . . . . . . . . . . . . . . . . . . . 127

Pawan Sharma, Swarndeep Singh, and Arghya Pal

**13 Public Health Aspects of Dhat Syndrome** . . . . . . . . . . . . . . . . . . . . . . 137
Russell Kabir, Madhini Sivasubramanian, Sumayea Binte Mizan, and Ali Davod Parsa

**14 Current Research and Gaps in Dhat Syndrome** . . . . . . . . . . . . . . . . . 151
Nishtha Laspal and Siddharth Sarkar

**15 Dhat Syndrome: A Fact or Myth** . . . . . . . . . . . . . . . . . . . . . . . . . . . . . . 163
Mohammad Muntasir Maruf, Tamkeen Saleem, and S. M. Yasir Arafat

# About the Editors

**Sujita Kumar Kar** is currently working as an Additional Professor of Psychiatry at King George's Medical University, Lucknow, Uttar Pradesh, India. He is the editor in chief of *Indian Journal of Health, Sexuality and Culture*. He is also the editorial board member and reviewer of various national and international journals. He had written 42 book chapters and more than 350 articles in various national and international journals, and made 70 presentations in various national and international conferences. His research interests include brain stimulation, neuropsychiatry, and suicide prevention.

**S. M. Yasir Arafat** is currently working as an Assistant Professor of Psychiatry at Enam Medical College and Hospital, Dhaka, Bangladesh. He focuses on the epidemiological aspects of mental disorders and human behaviors. He completed MD in Psychiatry from Bangabandhu Sheikh Mujib Medical University, Dhaka, and MBBS from the Dhaka Medical College, Dhaka, Bangladesh. He also did an MPH in Health Economics and MBA in Marketing. Dr. Arafat has (co)authored more than 300 peer-reviewed articles and book chapters and (co)edited several books. He has been included in the global 2% researcher list in 2021 and 2022.

**Vikas Menon** is currently working at the Jawaharlal Institute of Postgraduate Medical Education and Research (JIPMER), Puducherry, India. He completed his postgraduate training in Psychiatry in 2008 from JIPMER. His research interests primarily lie in understanding the biological aspects as well as the long-term course and outcomes of mood disorders and suicide. In particular, he is interested in harnessing low-cost technology to reduce the treatment gap in psychiatry and support traditional interventions to improve clinical outcomes. He has published over 300 peer-reviewed research papers in scientific journals, 16 book chapters in edited volumes, and edited a book on Bipolar Disorders. His work has been funded by both national and international funding agencies. He is presently the Deputy Editor of *Indian Journal of Psychiatry*, Chief Associate Editor of the *Indian Journal of Psychological Medicine*, and Editor of the *International Journal of Advanced Medical and Health Research.*

# List of Figures

Fig. 1.1 Phenomenological and nosological overlap between Dhat syndrome and other mental disorders . . . . . . . . . . . . . . . . . . 10
Fig. 4.1 Formation of semen according to ayurveda and seven essential elements of the Human Body . . . . . . . . . . . . . . . . . . . . . . . . . . . . 39
Fig. 4.2 Formation of semen cascade. Adapted from Sharma and Chaudhary (2014)) . . . . . . . . . . . . . . . . . . . . . . . . . . . . . . . 39
Fig. 5.1 Etiological model of Dhat syndrome . . . . . . . . . . . . . . . . . . . . . . 52
Fig. 6.1 The biopsychosocial model of sexual response (Clark and Watson 1991) . . . . . . . . . . . . . . . . . . . . . . . . . . . . . . . 64
Fig. 8.1 Clinical features of Dhat syndrome . . . . . . . . . . . . . . . . . . . . . . . 87
Fig. 11.1 Cognitive model for Dhat syndrome (Gupta 2017) . . . . . . . . . . . . 121
Fig. 13.1 Prevention of Dhat syndrome . . . . . . . . . . . . . . . . . . . . . . . . . . . . . 141
Fig. 13.2 Combined strategy for preventing Dhat syndrome . . . . . . . . . . . . . 143
Fig. 14.1 Schematic representation of phenomenological aspects of Dhat syndrome . . . . . . . . . . . . . . . . . . . . . . . . . . . . . . . . . . . . 152

# List of Tables


Table 1.1 Studies of the phenomenology of Dhat syndrome .............. 6
Table 2.1 Symptoms in patients of Dhat Syndromes (Deb and Balhara 2013; Dhungana et al. 2017; Gautham et al. 2008; Grover et al. 2015). .................... 23
Table 2.2 Summary of presenting symptoms by patients with Dhat syndrome (Balhara 2011; Bhatia 1999; Bhatia and Malik 1991; Chadda and Ahuja 1990; Deb and Balhara 2013; Jadhav 2004) ...................... 24
Table 2.3 Comparison of symptomatology of male and female Dhat Syndrome (Avasthi et al. 2012; Bhatti and Fikree 2002; Grover et al. 2014; Patel et al. 2005, 2008; Singh et al. 2001; Trollope-Kumar 2001) .................................. 24
Table 4.1 Common signs and symptoms of Dhat Syndrome across the sexes .................................... 43
Table 6.1 Common symptoms associated with Dhat syndrome (Grover et al. 2015a, b; Jhanjee et al. 2011; Udina et al. 2013). . 63
Table 6.2 Comorbidity in Dhat syndrome (Deb and Balhara 2013; Winokur and Coryell 1992; Grover et al. 2015a, b). ........... 63
Table 8.1 Common symptoms observed in patients with Dhat syndrome (Grover et al. 2014a, b, 2016a, b; Kar et al. 2021; Prakash et al. 2016; Strong et al. 2022) .................... 88
Table 8.2 Assessment for patients with Dhat syndrome ................ 90
Table 11.1 Differential diagnoses of semen loss/leakage (Ronald 2018) . . 118
Table 12.1 Common symptoms reported among women with Female Dhat Syndrome ............................ 131
Table 14.1 Research gaps and the way forward for Dhat syndrome ...... 158
Table 15.1 Commonly available myths and facts regarding Dhat syndrome ...................................... 171

# Chapter 1
# The Phenomenology of Dhat Syndrome

**Ravi Philip Rajkumar**

## 1.1 Introduction

The term "phenomenology" has its origins in philosophy, where it refers to a tradition or school of thought founded by Edmund Husserl. Phenomenology can be defined as "the study of the structures of experience or consciousness….as experienced from the first-person point of view" (Smith 2013). Psychiatric disorders are characterized by disturbances in the contents of consciousness and experience, including thought, emotions, perception, volition, memory and planned action, all of which are experienced and reported in the first person by individual patients (Madeira et al. 2019). For this reason, the phenomenological approach has been influential in describing and classifying the symptoms of psychiatric disorders (Jacob 2012; Englander 2016). In the fields of psychiatry and psychology, the terms "phenomenology", "psychopathology", and "descriptive psychopathology" are used interchangeably to describe the application of phenomenology to the signs and symptoms of mental illness (Telles-Correia and Sampaio, 2016). This field is a key component of training in psychiatry and related disciplines, and can be considered the "language of psychiatry" (Etxeandia-Pradera et al. 2021). Because it attempts to understand the unusual and often distressing experiences of patients from their perspective, using both empathy and a scientific approach, phenomenology serves as a bridge between the "art" and the "science" of psychiatry (Jacob 2012). It can improve both the quality of the therapeutic relationship and the classification of specific symptoms of mental illness (Madeira et al. 2019).

R. P. Rajkumar (✉)
Department of Psychiatry, Jawaharlal Institute of Postgraduate Medical Education and Research (JIPMER), Puducherry, India

© The Author(s), under exclusive license to Springer Nature Singapore Pte Ltd. 2024

S. K. Kar et al. (eds.), *Dhat Syndrome*,
https://doi.org/10.1007/978-981-99-8870-9_1

Dhat syndrome was first described in the psychiatric literature by Wig (1960), and this initial description was elaborated upon in a subsequent paper by Malhotra and Wig (1975). The original description of this condition combined phenomenological and cultural points of view. Dhat syndrome was seen as a "culture-bound symptom complex" that involved specific phenomena—anxiety and hypochondriasis—related to loss of semen, which was culturally viewed as an "elixir of life" or *dhatu* (Malhotra and Wig 1975). The first study explicitly designed to study the phenomenology of Dhat syndrome was carried out by Behere and Natraj in a sample of 50 men from Varanasi. This study found that 38% of patients reported anxiety related to semen loss, while 46% reported hypochondriacal concerns related to this theme. Several patients also reported somatic preoccupations, though this was not quantified by the authors. Two-thirds of these patients reported a complete resolution of symptoms when treated over a year (Behere and Natraj 1984). Subsequently, several studies have examined the psychological phenomena that characterize Dhat syndrome and their demographic and clinical correlates and have called attention to its existence outside the Indian subcontinent (Jadhav 2007; Menendez et al. 2013). Some researchers have identified a similar condition in women, characterized by anxiety and somatic preoccupations related to non-pathological vaginal discharge (Chaturvedi et al. 1993). This chapter aims to summarize the existing evidence related to the phenomenology of Dhat syndrome and to explore the implications of specific phenomena for the diagnosis and management of this condition.

## 1.2 Form and Content in the Phenomenology of Dhat Syndrome

An important distinction to be made when analyzing psychiatric disorders from a phenomenological perspective is between *form* and *content*. This is sometimes referred to as the "form-content dichotomy" (Khanna and Channabasavanna 1988; Markova and Berrios 1994; Rajesh and Jacob 2004). *Form* refers to broad categories of mental phenomena that can be reliably distinguished from each other, and that have value in differentiating between specific disorders. *Content* refers to the theme or topic that the specific phenomenon addresses or "contains". This distinction can be illustrated through the following example:

> Patient A reports a belief that a group of scientists from another country is stealing semen from him while sleeping. He interprets normal physiological phenomena, such as early morning erections, as being related to this, and claims that this is because they want to weaken him and use his spermatozoa for genetic experiments in a secret laboratory. On the other hand, patient B reports repeated preoccupations with semen loss during nocturnal emissions. He complains of various physical symptoms, such as fatigue and back pain, which he attributes to loss of semen.

In this case, the *content* of both patients' psychopathology is broadly similar, dealing with the loss of semen. However, the *form* is different—the first patient has a delusion, while the second has a somatic preoccupation related to semen loss. In

Western psychiatric practice, there is an unspoken assumption that *form* is largely biologically determined, while *content* is influenced by cultural and social factors (Littlewood 1996). Modern psychiatric nosology largely relies on the *form* to distinguish between specific disorders (Rajesh and Jacob 2004). However, ignoring the *content* of psychopathology can lead to an emphasis on artificially constructed criteria and categories and a neglect of the individual patient's specific problems and cultural background. Andreasen (2007) has referred to this as "the death of phenomenology". When studying Dhat syndrome, it is essential to avoid this potential pitfall, and to consider both the form and the content of the subjective experiences reported by patients suffering from this disorder.

The original description of Dhat syndrome (Malhotra and Wig 1975; Behere and Natraj 1984; Chadda and Ahuja 1990) identified phenomena considered to be specific to the disorder in terms of both form and content. In these reports, abnormalities of *form* included hypochondriasis and somatic preoccupations. Abnormalities in *content* were centred on the theme of loss of semen either while passing urine, through nocturnal emission, or through sexual activities that were considered culturally inappropriate (i.e., masturbation, pre- or extra-marital intercourse). The importance of this distinction was underlined in a study by Singh (1985) involving 50 male patients with a history of sexual dysfunction. Though 31 (62%) of these patients reported concerns related to semen loss, only 11 (22%) could be diagnosed as having Dhat syndrome. In a similar study of patients with a presenting complaint of semen or "Dhat" loss, only 13.5% (7 of 52 patients) could be diagnosed to have Dhat syndrome—the others received diagnoses of depression, anxiety disorder, or psychogenic erectile dysfunction. In other words, even if the content of a patient's complaints includes the theme of semen loss, this is not sufficient to establish a diagnosis; the characteristic forms of psychopathology, namely anxiety, hypochondriacal ideas and/or somatic preoccupations specifically related to this content, should also be present. Symptoms with "Dhat content" or a "Dhat theme" can be seen in other disorders, particularly depression (Singh 1985; Prakash 2013), and a careful evaluation of both form and content is necessary for an accurate diagnosis. This point is of crucial importance both in clinical practice and in research and will be discussed in more detail when examining the cultural basis of "Dhat content" and reviewing the existing literature on the phenomenology of Dhat syndrome.

## 1.3 The Cultural Roots of "Dhat" as Content in Phenomenology

As noted above, culture can have a marked influence on the content of psychopathology, regardless of its form. For example, a social anxiety disorder in North American or European patients is associated with fears of scrutiny or negative evaluation by others, while the same disorder in Japan may be associated with a fear of offending others through one's appearance or behaviour. This difference in the content of the patient's thoughts reflects differing cultural values and orientations, such as the cultural dimension of individualism-collectivism (Clarvit et al. 1996; Matsunaga et al. 2001). Similarly, the content of obsessions in obsessive-compulsive disorder can vary significantly across cultures (Akhtar et al. 1978). To evaluate how culture influences the content of psychopathology in Dhat syndrome, it is important to understand certain culture-specific beliefs related to health and illness that are specific to the Indian sub-continent. In Ayurveda, a traditional system of medicine whose origins can be traced back to the Vedic era, health is seen as arising from the balance between seven essential elements or *dhatus* in the human body: blood, muscle, semen (*sukra*), bone, marrow, fat, and fluid from digested food. In the *Charaka Samhita*, one of the foundational texts of Ayurvedic medicine, a deficiency of *sukra* is said to be associated with symptoms such as fatigue, lack of energy, and erectile dysfunction. However, this text does not specifically attribute any specific "disease" or "syndrome" to semen loss *per se.* (Behere et al. 1991; Money et al. 1991; Jadhav 2004; Prakash et al. 2014). The term "dhat" is a modification or corruption of the Sanskrit word *dhatu*, and is something of a misnomer, as *dhatu* refers to any essential element and not specifically to semen (Jadhav 2004). This ancient belief survives today in a modified or distorted form, both as a "folk" explanation for weakness or male sexual dysfunction and as an explanatory model for ill-health proposed by practitioners of indigenous medicine and in the media (Lakhani et al. 2001; Kattimani et al. 2013). Such beliefs have been documented even in individuals who have received a formal education in allopathic medicine. In a study involving male medical students who had passed their final examinations and were undergoing their internship, over 50% believed that "semen loss" could lead to physical weakness, and over 75% reported that it could lead to a reduction in penile size (Mangot et al. 2017). However, it would not be correct to diagnose these young men with "Dhat syndrome". In other words, men can present with concerns or beliefs related to semen loss in the absence of any mental or physical disorder, or connection with a variety of physical and psychological disorders, including erectile dysfunction, depression, and even HIV/AIDS (Mumford 1996; Lakhani et al. 2001; Manjula et al. 2003). In such cases, a diagnosis of "Dhat syndrome" would again be inappropriate: rather, these individuals are using a culturally accepted explanatory model for a specific condition that should be treated in its own right. The diagnosis of Dhat syndrome should be reserved for patients with somatic concerns or hypochondriacal ideas (health anxiety), occurring in the presence of medically unexplained symptoms such as fatigue or bodily pain, and in the absence of other syndromal diagnoses such as depression, anxiety disorders or psychosis. Failure to make the distinction between "dhat" as culturally determined thought content, and "Dhat syndrome" as specifically described by Wig, can lead to errors both in patient care and in the formulation of appropriate research questions about this disorder (Prakash and Mandal 2015).

A culturally conditioned phenomenon that is closely related to Dhat syndrome, but distinct from it, is masturbatory guilt (Prakash 2013; Aneja et al. 2015). Though masturbation is a common form of sexual behaviour observed across countries and cultures, it is often viewed as sinful, unhealthy, or socially unacceptable (War and Albert 2013; Vivekanandan et al. 2019). Such attitudes and beliefs can act synergistically with the beliefs related to semen loss described in the previous paragraph in two ways:

- Patients with Dhat syndrome may attribute their semen loss to excessive masturbation;
- Patients with another medical or psychiatric condition, such as erectile dysfunction or depression, can report concerns related to semen loss through masturbation as the "cause" for their disorder; in some cases, the disorder may even be viewed as a divinely inflicted "punishment" for the "sin" of masturbation (Vivekanandan et al. 2019).

Again, it is important to distinguish between the above cases, to avoid either an over- or an under-diagnosis of Dhat syndrome, and to provide effective psychological interventions in the latter case (Abdul Salam et al. 2012; Kar and Sarkar 2015).

It should be noted at this point that beliefs about the harmful consequences of semen loss or masturbation are not exclusive to Asian culture. As Sumathipala et al. (2004) pointed out, they have been reported in various ancient and modern cultures, ranging from ancient Greek and Roman civilization to modern industrialized societies such as Switzerland, the United Kingdom and the United States of America. It should also be noted that as cultural beliefs change over time, the occurrence of Dhat-related concerns and Dhat syndrome may vary in specific populations. For example, in countries with an influx of migrants sharing this belief, the incidence of such symptoms might increase over time; on the other hand, increased globalization and "Westernization" in Asian countries may lead to a decrease in their frequency (Halliburton 2005; Kar 2015). With this basic understanding of the link between culture and Dhat-related beliefs or ideas, it becomes easier to review both the common and rare psychopathological phenomena that have been reported in patients assigned a diagnosis of Dhat syndrome.

## 1.4 Empirical Research on the Phenomenology of Dhat Syndrome

### *1.4.1 Observational Studies*

After the initial reports described above, several researchers have helped to deepen our understanding of the form and content of psychopathology in Dhat syndrome. These studies are summarized in Table 1.1. The earliest studies (1984–1990), based on clinical observations, identified specific changes in affect (depressed mood and anxious mood) and thought (hypochondriacal ideas, somatic concerns, and depressive cognitions) in patients with Dhat syndrome. These studies also examined patients' thought content regarding semen loss which was commonly attributed to masturbation or pre-/extra-marital sexual activity. Chadda (1995) was the first to use a structured instrument, the Illness Behavior Questionnaire (Pilowsky et al. 1984),

**Table 1.1** Studies of the phenomenology of Dhat syndrome

| Study | Study sample size and characteristics | Instruments used | Findings related to form | Findings related to content |
|---|---|---|---|---|
| **Studies in male patients** | | | | |
| Behere and Natraj (1984) | Male patients with a complaint of "Dhat" discharge, psychiatry OP setting ($n = 50$) | Clinical interview | Hypochondriacal and somatic preoccupations (frequency not reported). | Semen loss ascribed to masturbation (52%) or sexual relations outside marriage (30%) |
| Singh (1985) | Male patients with sexual dysfunction, psychiatry OP setting ($n = 50$) | Clinical interview | Somatic preoccupations related to semen loss (DS) in 62%. 63% of patients with DS had a depressed affect, 52% had an anxious affect, 13-26% had depressive cognitions | Attribution of sexual dysfunction to semen loss |
| Chadda and Ahuja (1990) | Male patients with a complaint of "Dhat" discharge, psychiatry OP setting ($n = 52$) | Clinical interview | Only 13% of patients with a complaint of "Dhat" discharge met criteria for DS as specified in earlier literature | N/A |
| Chadda (1995) | Men with DS ($n = 66$) and healthy controls ($n = 50$), general hospital OP setting | IBQ | Patients with DS scored higher on the hypochondriasis and anxiety/depression scales of the IBQ than controls | N/A |
| Grover et al. (2016a) | Men with DS ($n = 780$) from 15 hospitals across India | DSQ | Depressed mood in 68%; lack of interest in activities or anhedonia in 64% | Semen loss attributed to masturbation (55%), sexual dreams (47%), or diet (37%); semen loss described as occurring during nocturnal emission (60%) or while passing stools (60%) |
| Prakash et al. (2016) | Men with DS, community clinic setting ($n = 100$) | DDSS, HAM-A, HAM-D | Anxiety or worry in 95-99%; somatic concerns in 99%; ideas of hopelessness related to treatment in 97%. Factor analysis of health beliefs yielded three dimensions (salience, coherence, strength); factor analysis of associated symptoms also yielded three dimensions (loss of vitality, preoccupation, and retardation-arousal) | Semen loss is described as occurring during passage or urine or stools (75%), nocturnal emission (73%) or masturbation (49%) |

**Table 1.1** (continued)

| Study | Study sample size and characteristics | Instruments used | Findings related to form | Findings related to content |
|---|---|---|---|---|
| Prakash et al. (2018) | Men with DS, hospital OP settings ($n = 12$) | Qualitative; FGD | Beliefs not amounting to a delusional level about the "precious" nature of semen and of a link between semen loss and ill-health; anxious affect reported by 50%; somatic concerns reported by all subjects | Semen loss attributed to "excessive sexual stimulation" (67%) or masturbation (20%) |
| **Studies in female patients** | | | | |
| Grover et al. (2016b) | Women with depressive or somatic symptoms related to normal vaginal discharge, psychiatry OP setting ($n = 26$) | SAFED | Somatic or hypochondriacal concerns were reported in 54%; depressed mood and depressive cognitions in 19% | Discharge attributed to urinary or genital infection (34–42%) Discharge is described as occurring unrelated to a specific situation (75%), or related to menstruation (39%), sexual arousal (39%), or passage or urine or stools (34%) |
| Mehra et al. (2021) | Women with normal vaginal discharge, gynaecology OP setting ($n = 69$) | SAFED | N/A | Discharge attributed to diet (75%), infection (64%) or constipation (49%); discharge described as occurring unrelated to any specific situation (78%), while passing urine (46%), or during sexual dreams (46%) |
| Joshi et al. (2022) | Women with distress related to normal vaginal discharge, gynaecology OP setting ($n = 70$) | HADS Somatic symptom assessment adapted from PHQ-15 | Somatic concerns were reported in 67%; significant depression in 19% and anxiety in 10%; subclinical depression in 23% and anxiety in 26% | Discharge attributed to menstruation (59%), infection (58%), or diet (36%); discharge described as occurring unrelated to any specific situation (84%), during sexual arousal (20%) or passage of stools (20%) |

**Abbreviations:** *DDSS* Dhat Disorder Severity Scale, Dhat syndrome, *DSQ* Dhat Syndrome Questionnaire, *FGD* focus group discussions, *HADS* Hospital Anxiety and Depression Scale, *HAM-A* Hamilton Rating Scale for Anxiety, *HAM-D* Hamilton Rating Scale for Depression, *IBQ* Illness Behavior Questionnaire, *N/A* not applicable (i.e., the specific domain was not evaluated in the study under consideration), *OP* outpatient, *PHQ* Patient Health Questionnaire, *SAFED* Scale for Assessment of Female Dhat syndrome to compare patients with Dhat syndrome and healthy controls. This study confirmed the specific associations of hypochondriacal ideas and changes in mood (depressed or anxious affect) with this syndrome.

In 2016, two groups of researchers conducted more in-depth examinations of the phenomenology of Dhat syndrome. In the first study, Grover et al. (2016b) developed the *Dhat Syndrome Questionnaire (DSQ)* and administered it to 780 male patients from 15 centres in India. They found that depressed mood was found in over 60% of patients with Dhat syndrome. When examining thought content, they found that semen loss was most commonly attributed to masturbation, sexual dreams, or dietary habits, and was often considered to occur during nocturnal emissions or the passage of stools. In the second, Prakash et al. (2016) developed a similar instrument, the *Dhat Disorder Severity Scale (DDSS)* and applied it to 100 patients attending a community health centre. They also performed factor analyses of the DDSS items, identifying three dimensions related to beliefs about Dhat (salience of the belief, its coherence, and its intensity) and three dimensions of associated symptoms, which corresponded roughly to loss of energy, anxiety, and depression. Thought contents related to semen loss were similar to those reported in the Grover et al. study. Prakash et al. (2018) also conducted the first structured qualitative study of the phenomenology of Dhat syndrome, involving focus group discussions with 12 patients. The themes that emerged through these discussions were: a culturally conditioned belief in the "precious" or "vital" nature of semen; an attribution of semen loss to "excessive sexual stimulation" or masturbation; associations of semen loss with weakness, anxiety and body pain, but not depression; and a belief that symptoms were physical in origin. Based on this data, Prakash et al. formulated a tentative set of diagnostic guidelines for Dhat syndrome.

Though "female Dhat syndrome" has been described in several case reports and series (Singh et al. 2001; Kar and Singh 2017), systematic studies of its phenomenology were conducted only from 2016 onwards. In a pioneering study, Grover et al. (2016b) adapted the DSQ for use in women and renamed it the *Scale for Assessment of Female Dhat Syndrome (SAFED)*. When they administered the SAFED to women with suspected female Dhat syndrome, it was found that somatic and hypochondriacal ideas were reported by half of the patients, but depressive symptoms were observed in less than 20% of them. Examination of thought content in this sample found that discharge was most commonly ascribed to urinary or genital tract infection, and was most commonly considered to occur spontaneously, or in relation to menstruation, sexual arousal, or micturition/defecation. Mehra et al. (2021) used the SAFED in a larger sample of women seeking help in a gynaecology clinic. This study focused mainly on thought content related to vaginal discharge, which women attributed to dietary habits, infection or constipation, and described as occurring similarly to the women studied by Grover and colleagues. The most recent study of female Dhat syndrome used specific rating scales for depression, anxiety and somatic symptoms instead of the SAFED (Joshi et al. 2022). In this study, somatic concerns were again found to be twice to thrice as common as depression or anxiety; thoughts regarding the causes or means of passage of vaginal discharge were similar to those reported in the earlier studies.

### 1.4.2 Case Reports

Despite their lower value in terms of the quality of evidence, case reports are useful in highlighting unusual presentations or phenomena related to Dhat syndrome. Ghosh and Chowdhury (2020) described a case where Dhat syndrome co-existed with concerns about shrinkage of the penis, similar to the culture-bound syndrome of *Koro*; however, this patient also had comorbid obsessive-compulsive disorder which may have influenced his symptomatology. Darshan et al. (2014) reported a case of comorbid pornography addiction and Dhat syndrome, in which concerns about potency and seminal quantity/quality were seen in addition to typical thoughts about semen loss. This patient also reported prominent masturbatory guilt, which has been reported both with and without Dhat syndrome in male patients from India (Aneja et al. 2015). Some patients present with unusual beliefs relating to the mode of semen loss, including through saliva and perspiration (Arafat et al. 2021), or through the anus (Balhara and Goel 2012; Kar and Singh 2015). In these cases, the associated clinical features were typical of Dhat syndrome. In contrast, Mitra et al. (2017) reported an otherwise typical case of Dhat syndrome in an adolescent male, but with an unusual overvalued idea regarding "bone loss" due to nocturnal emissions. In some cases, the distress associated with semen loss and its feared consequences has been associated with bizarre behaviours, such as ingestion of one's own semen (Agarwal et al. 2022) or genital self-mutilation (Maheshwari et al. 2022). Finally, a case of Dhat syndrome "by proxy" has been reported in a middle-aged man, who presented with somatic and hypochondriacal concerns related to his adolescent son who was experiencing nocturnal emissions (Hafi et al. 2022). In this case, the child did not present with any symptoms or concerns, and treatment was required only for the father.

## 1.5 A Synthesis of the Available Evidence on the Phenomenology of Dhat Syndrome

A careful examination of the research studies and case reports discussed above yields certain common themes. In terms of form, Dhat syndrome involves disturbances in both thought and affect. The most frequently reported disturbance of thought involves thought content, and centres on ideas related to semen loss and its deleterious consequences which are held with a high, but not unshakeable, degree of conviction. Phenomenologically, such ideas would be characterized as *overvalued ideas*. The concept of the overvalued idea was first introduced by Wernicke and refers to ideas which are not delusions but which are associated with a strong negative emotional "tone" and "dominate the sufferer's life" (McKenna 1984; Mullen and Linscott 2010). Overvalued ideas can be seen in a variety of psychiatric disorders, including obsessive-compulsive disorder (OCD), anorexia nervosa (AN), and hypochondriasis (Kozak and Foa 1994; Mountjoy et al. 2014). In all these conditions, they are strongly associated with an anxious affect, which is also seen in Dhat syndrome. However, Dhat syndrome can be clearly distinguished from these conditions: it is not associated with the particular repetitive, intrusive and ego-dystonic thoughts seen in OCD, it does not involve significant disturbances in body image as seen in AN, and it does not involve fears of a specific, life-threatening disease as seen in hypochondriasis.

Apart from overvalued ideas, many patients with Dhat syndrome report somatic or anxious preoccupations related to physical and sexual health, similar to those seen in bodily distress disorders (Henningsen et al. 2018). These somatic concerns are not held as firmly as overvalued ideas but are also associated with negative affect states such as anxiety and depression. They differ from those seen in bodily distress disorders in that they are associated with an explanatory model involving semen loss (Kar and Sarkar 2015; Grover et al. 2016a). An unanswered question in Dhat syndrome, but one that is crucial from a phenomenological perspective, is whether these ideas are primary, or whether they are secondary to another psychological phenomenon, such as a mood state (Rajkumar and Bharadwaj 2014) or a misinterpretation of bodily sensations (Abramowitz 2005). Based on these considerations, and the factor-analytic research of Prakash et al. (2016), it can be stated—provisionally—that Dhat syndrome can be best understood as a heterogeneous construct, involving symptoms across various dimensions (somatic concerns and symptoms, anxiety, and depression) and variations in the intensity and extension of the ideas related to semen loss, ranging from anxious cognitions to overvalued ideas. These symptoms overlap with those of other psychiatric syndromes, but should not be seen as identical with them (Fig. 1.1).

It is also important to distinguish between Dhat-related thought content, which can occur in a variety of syndromes (e.g., a patient with depression who has ideas of guilt related to sexual activity and semen loss, in which case the depressed mood is the primary psychopathology), and the specific constellation of changes in thought

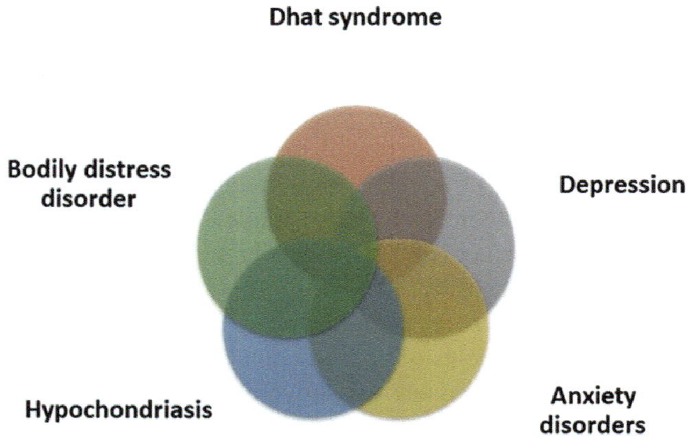


**Fig. 1.1** Phenomenological and nosological overlap between Dhat syndrome and other mental disorders

and mood that best characterizes the Dhat syndrome (Prakash et al. 2018). Finally, unusual presentations pertaining either to the mode of semen loss or its consequences can be reported in some patients; based on the available case reports, such cases can still be diagnosed and treated as Dhat syndrome.

Research into the phenomenology of Dhat-like symptoms and syndromes in women is still at an early stage (Table 1.1). The available evidence suggests that it shares some features with "male" Dhat syndrome, such as somatic concerns, a belief that loss of vaginal fluid can cause ill-health, and the presence of a depressed or anxious affect (Grover et al. 2016b; Joshi et al. 2022). However, there are also important differences: women frequently report spontaneous passage of vaginal discharge without any external trigger and often relate their symptoms to gender-specific factors such as genitourinary infection, female sexual arousal or menstruation. These differences suggest that this condition merits further study, both in terms of phenomenology and in terms of its relationship to cultural beliefs regarding femininity, female sexuality and reproductive health (Chandra et al. 1993; Grover et al. 2014; Tripathi et al. 2021).

## 1.6 Implications of Phenomenology for the Nosology of Dhat Syndrome

While it is beyond the scope of this chapter to discuss the current concepts and controversies surrounding the nosology of Dhat syndrome (Prakash and Mandal 2014; Arafat 2017), certain key findings from phenomenological research can help in resolving these controversies. Some authors (Mumford 1996; Dhikav et al. 2007) have suggested that Dhat syndrome is simply "a culturally appropriate manifestation of depression". However, the available phenomenological evidence does not entirely support this contention, as depression is not an invariable concomitant of overvalued ideas or preoccupations related to semen loss (Singh 1985; Grover et al. 2016a; Prakash et al. 2016, 2018). Moreover, male patients with depression in the Indian sub-continent do not frequently report ideas or beliefs related to Dhat (Grover et al. 2010), and factor analysis of symptoms in Dhat syndrome suggests that depressive symptoms are only one of the dimensions of this disorder (Prakash et al. 2016). Similarly, though Dhat syndrome may share some phenomenological features with conditions such as hypochondriasis or somatization, there are certain features peculiar to it, such as overvalued ideas related to semen loss (and not to serious illness or symptoms *per se*) and an absence of the quasi-obsessional, reassurance-seeking quality of symptoms seen in hypochondriasis (Abramowitz 2005).

It is too early to conclude that Dhat syndrome is simply a culturally conditioned variant of another syndrome, such as depression, bodily distress disorder or hypochondriasis (Prakash and Mandal 2015), though these hypotheses remain viable and should be tested through careful analyses of patients' reported symptoms and the cultural context in which they occur. It is most useful to view this syndrome as a "biocultural patterned illness experience", as in the case of neurasthenia in China, which cannot be shoe-horned into a single existing category (Kleinman 1982), but whose symptoms overlap with those of other recognized syndromes (Fig. 1.1). The diagnostic criteria proposed by some Indian researchers (Prakash et al. 2016, 2018) are a valuable, phenomenologically-based starting point from which the proper nosological status of Dhat syndrome, its symptom dimensions, and its diagnostic stability can be adequately investigated. Likewise, the use of dimensional, scientifically validated systems such as the *Research Domain Criteria (RDoC)* can be used to link biology, culture and phenomenology in Dhat syndrome and deepen our understanding of its symptom dimensions and its proper place in psychiatric nosology (Prakash et al. 2016; Hasratian et al. 2022), and can validate existing findings on the dimensions of Dhat syndrome. Similar considerations should be taken into account when linking phenomenology to the nosology of Dhat syndrome in women.

## 1.7 Implications of Phenomenology for the Treatment of Dhat Syndrome

There is no single well-established or evidence-based treatment for Dhat syndrome. Both pharmacological and psychological approaches have been used in case reports and series. Though it cannot substitute for evidence from controlled clinical trials, phenomenological research can serve as a valuable guide when selecting treatments based on a given patient's reported changes in mood and thought. For example, patients with Dhat syndrome and a prominent depressed affect may respond better to antidepressants such as fluoxetine (Dhikav et al. 2008), while those with anxiety may benefit from the short-term use of anxiolytics (Prakash 2007). Similarly, variations in thought content can guide and inform psychotherapeutic approaches; if the therapist does not consider the patient's ideas and concerns, patients are likely to drop out of therapy (Bhatia et al. 1989). Likewise, simple sex education is insufficient to treat established cases of Dhat syndrome (Abdul Salam et al. 2012). Cognitive and behavioural techniques, often used in the management of somatization or hypochondriasis, can be successfully adapted to managing Dhat syndrome. These methods can be tailored to the specific form and content of an individual's ideas related to Dhat (Kar and Singh, 2016, 2017). For example, a patient with overvalued ideas about the consequences of semen loss can be treated through exposure to cues or triggers that evoke health anxiety, followed by prevention of reassurance-seeking or safety behaviours, targeted education about normal sexual physiology, and identifying and correcting erroneous beliefs or interpretations. This approach would be similar to the techniques used in hypochondriasis (Visser and Bouman 1992; Abramowitz et al. 2002). On the other hand, a patient with predominantly physical symptoms and somatic concerns can benefit from approaches similar to those used in somatoform disorders. These include relaxation techniques or yoga (for body pain related to semen-loss anxiety), graded involvement in activities (to address complaints of fatigue or weakness due to semen loss), and identifying and addressing dysfunctional cognitions related to semen loss, sexuality or physical health (Allen et al. 2001).

## 1.8 Conclusions

Phenomenology remains a valuable approach to the study of Dhat syndrome, from both clinical and research perspectives. Clinicians working in the Indian subcontinent, or in other cultures where they are likely to encounter this syndrome, should be aware of the fundamental phenomenology of this syndrome—overvalued ideas and somatic preoccupations related to semen loss and its consequences, and associated changes in mood—as well as the range of ideas that patients report regarding the causes and routes of semen loss, and their cultural origins. They should also be aware of the existence of an analogous condition in women and should liaise with other medical disciplines, such as urology and gynaecology, which may serve as the first point of contact for these patients. This will ensure that these patients receive an appropriate diagnosis and timely treatment. When treating Dhat syndrome, both pharmacological and psychological therapies should target the specific phenomena reported by them, such as serotonin reuptake inhibitors for depressed mood and specific behavioural techniques for hypochondriacal ideas or somatic preoccupations. Research into the phenomenology of Dhat syndrome is at a crucial stage, as the development of structured instruments and questionnaires for use in both men and women can lead to a better understanding of symptom dimensions or domains in this disorder through factor or principal components analysis of large data sets. Linking phenomenology to studies of the biological and sociocultural correlates of Dhat syndrome can help to resolve controversies about its nosological status, and will lead to the development of better treatment strategies.

## References

Abdul Salam KP, Sharma MP, Prakash O. Development of cognitive-behavioral therapy intervention for patients with Dhat syndrome. Indian J Psychiatry. 2012;54(4):367–74. https://doi.org/10.4103/0019-5545.104826.

Abramowitz JS. Hypochondriasis: conceptualization, treatment, and relationship to obsessive compulsive disorder. Ann Clin Psychiatry. 2005;17(4):211–7. https://doi.org/10.1080/10401230500295339.

Abramowitz JS, Schwartz SA, Whiteside SP. A contemporary conceptual model of hypochondriasis. Mayo Clin Proc. 2002;77:1323–30. https://doi.org/10.4065/77.12.1323.

Agarwal AK, Bagewadi V, Das S, Moirangthem S. Recycling of semen: a rare phenomenon in Dhat syndrome. Psychiatr Danub. 2022;34(2):313–4. https://doi.org/10.24869/psyd.2022.313.

Akhtar S, Wig NN, Varma VK, Pershad D, Verma SK. Socio-cultural and clinical determinants of symptomatology in obsessional neurosis. Int J Soc Psychiatry. 1978;24(3):157–62. https://doi.org/10.1177/002076407802400301.

Allen LA, Woolfolk RL, Lehrer PM, Gara MA, Escobar JI. Cognitive behavior therapy for somatization disorder: a preliminary investigation. J Behav Ther Exp Psychiatry. 2001;32:53–62. https://doi.org/10.1016/s0005-7916(01)00020-9.
Andreasen NC. DSM and the death of phenomenology in America: an example of unintended consequences. Schizophr Bull. 2007;33(1):108–12. https://doi.org/10.1093/schbul/sbl054.
Aneja J, Grover S, Avasthi A, Mahajan S, Pokhrel P, Triveni D. Can masturbatory guilt lead to severe psychopathology: a case series. Indian J Psychol Med. 2015;37(1):81–6. https://doi.org/10.4103/0253-7176.150848.
Arafat SMY. Dhat syndrome: culture bound, separate entity, or removed. J Behav Health. 2017;6(3):147–50. https://doi.org/10.5455/jbh.20170123102726.
Arafat SMY, Mondal F, Ghimire S. A 47-year-old man passing putrid semen through saliva and sweat: a case of Dhat syndrome. J Gen Fam Med. 2021;23:177–9. https://doi.org/10.1002/jgf2.513.
Balhara YPS, Goel R. An unusual presentation of Dhat syndrome. J Neuropsychiatry Clin Neurosci. 2012;24(3):E19–20. https://doi.org/10.1176/appi.neuropsych.11070153.
Behere PB, Natraj GS. Dhat syndrome: the phenomenology of a culture bound sex neurosis of the orient. Indian J Psychiatry. 1984;26(1):76–8.
Behere PS, Wig NN, Behere M. Ancient Indian concept of Dhat syndrome: a cultural bound sex neurosis of the Orient. Indian J Psychol Med. 1991;14(1):85–7. https://doi.org/10.1177/0975156419910114.
Bhatia MS, Bohra N, Malik SC. 'Dhat' syndrome—a useful clinical entity. Indian J Dermatol. 1989;34(2):32–41.
Chadda RK. Dhat syndrome: is it a distinct clinical entity? A study of illness behaviour characteristics. Acta Psychiatr Scand. 1995;91(2):136–9. https://doi.org/10.1111/j.1600-0447.1995.tb09754.x.
Chadda RK, Ahuja N. Dhat syndrome. A sex neurosis of the Indian subcontinent. Br J Psychiatry. 1990;156:577–9. https://doi.org/10.1192/bjp.156.4.577.
Chandra PS, Isaac MK, Sudarshan CY, Rao S. Is there a female Dhat syndrome? NIMHANS J. 1993;11(2):89–93.
Chaturvedi SK, Chandra PS, Isaac MK, Sudarshan CY. Somatization misattributed to non-pathological vaginal discharge. J Psychosom Res. 1993;37(6):575–9. https://doi.org/10.1016/0022-3999(93)90051-g.
Clarvit SR, Schneier FR, Liebowitz MR. The offensive subtype of Taijin-kyofu-sho in New York City: the phenomenology and treatment of a social anxiety disorder. J Clin Psychiatry. 1996;57(11):523–7. https://doi.org/10.4088/jcp.v57n1104.
Darshan MS, Rao TSS, Manickam S, Tandon A, Ram D. A case report of pornography addiction with dhat syndrome. Indian J Psychiatry. 2014;56(4):385–7. https://doi.org/10.4103/0019-5545.146536.
Dhikav V, Aggarwal N, Anand KS. Is Dhat syndrome a culturally appropriate manifestation of depression? Med Hypotheses. 2007;69(3):698. https://doi.org/10.1016/j.mehy.2007.01.019.
Dhikav V, Aggarwal N, Gupta S, Jadhavi R, Singh K. Depression in Dhat syndrome. J Sex Med. 2008;5(4):841–4. https://doi.org/10.1111/j.1743-6109.2007.00481.x.
Englander M. The phenomenological method in qualitative psychology and psychiatry. Int J Qual Stud Health Well Being. 2016;11:30682. https://doi.org/10.3402/qhw.v11.30682.
Etxeandia-Pradera J-I, Martinez-Uribe D, Bellver-Pradas F, Gonzalez-Piqueras J-C, Nacher J, Aguilar E-J. Training psychiatry residents in descriptive psychopathology: a systematic review. Psychopathology. 2021;54:1–17. https://doi.org/10.1159/000512791.
Ghosh S, Chowdhury AN. A case of two culture-bound syndromes (Koro and Dhat syndrome) coexisting with obsessive-compulsive disorder. Indian J Psychiatry. 2020;62(2):221–2. https://doi.org/10.4103/psychiatry.IndianJPsychiatry_298_19.
Grover S, Dutt A, Avasthi A. An overview of Indian research in depression. Indian J Psychiatry. 2010;52(Suppl. 1):S178–88. https://doi.org/10.4103/0019-5545.69231.

Grover S, Kate N, Avasthi A, Rajpal N, Umamaheswari V. Females too suffer from Dhat syndrome: a case series and revisit of the concept. Indian J Psychiatry. 2014;56(4):388–92. https://doi.org/10.4103/0019-5545.146537.

Grover S, Avasthi A, Gupta S, Dan A, Neogi R, Behere PB, Lakdawala B, Tripathi A, Chakraborthy K, Sinha V, Bhatia MS, Patjoshi A, Rao TSS, Rozatkar A. Phenomenology and beliefs of patients with Dhat syndrome: a nationwide multicentric study. Int J Soc Psychiatry. 2016a;62(1):57–66. https://doi.org/10.1177/0020764015591857.

Grover S, Avasthi A, Gupta S, Hazari N, Malhotra N. Do female patients with nonpathological vaginal discharge need the same evaluation as for Dhat syndrome in males? Indian J Psychiatry. 2016b;58(1):61–9. https://doi.org/10.4103/0019-5545.174376.

Hafi B, Uvais NA, Varughese A, Aysha S. Dhat syndrome by proxy: an underreported entity. Prim Care Companion CNS Disord. 2022;24(2):21cr02993. https://doi.org/10.4088/PCC.21cr02993.

Halliburton M. "Just some spirits": the erosion of spirit possession and the rise of "tension" in South India. Med Anthropol. 2005;24(2):111–44. https://doi.org/10.1080/01459740590933849.

Hasratian AM, Meuret AE, Chmielewski M, Ritz T. An examination of the RDoC negative valence systems domain constructs and the self-reports unit of analysis. Behav Ther. 2022;53(6):1092–108. https://doi.org/10.1016/j.beth.2022.04.009.

Henningsen P, Zipfel S, Sattel H, Creed F. Management of functional somatic syndromes and bodily distress. Psychother Psychosom. 2018;87(1):12–31. https://doi.org/10.1159/000484413.

Jacob KS. Psychiatric assessment and the art and science of clinical medicine. Indian J Psychiatry. 2012;54:184–7. https://doi.org/10.4103/0019-5545.99538.

Jadhav S. Dhat syndrome: a re-evaluation. Psychiatry. 2004;3(8):14–6. https://doi.org/10.1383/psyt.3.8.14.43399.

Jadhav S. Dhis and dhat: evidence of semen retention syndrome among white Britons. Anthropol Med. 2007;14(3):229–39. https://doi.org/10.1080/13648470701772770.

Joshi S, Tripathi A, Agarwal S, Singh N, Gupta B, Nischal A, Kar SK. Phenomenology, disability and sexual functioning in female Dhat syndrome: a study of tertiary care gynaecology outpatients. Gen Psychiatr. 2022;35:e100863. https://doi.org/10.1136/gpsych-2022-100863.

Kar SK. Dhat syndrome: will it reach a height or die soon? J Hum Reprod Sci. 2015;8:246. https://doi.org/10.4103/0974-1208.170421.

Kar SK, Sarkar S. Dhat syndrome: evolution of concept, current understanding, and need of an integrated approach. J Hum Reprod Sci. 2015;8(3):130–4. https://doi.org/10.4103/0974-1208.165143.

Kar SK, Singh A. Per-anal discharge: a new face of Dhat syndrome. J Hum Reprod Sci. 2015;8:245. https://doi.org/10.4103/0974-1208.170420.

Kar SK, Singh A. Person centered management approach for the Dhat syndrome. Int J Pers Cent Med. 2016;6(4):615. https://doi.org/10.5750/ijpcm.v6i4.615.

Kar SK, Singh A. Where lies the fault in diagnosing Dhat syndrome among females? Understanding through a case study. Indian J Psychol Med. 2017;39:506–8. https://doi.org/10.4103/0253-7176.211742.

Kattimani S, Menon V, Shrivastava MK. Is semen loss syndrome a psychological or physical illness? A case for conflict of interest. Indian J Psychol Med. 2013;35(4):420–2. https://doi.org/10.4103/0253-7176.122248.

Khanna S, Channabasavanna SM. Phenomenology of obsessions in obsessive-compulsive disorder. Psychopathology. 1988;21(1):12–8. https://doi.org/10.1159/000284534.

Kleinman A. Neurasthenia and depression: a study of somatization and culture in China. Cult Med Psychiatry. 1982;6(2):117–90. https://doi.org/10.1007/bf00051427.

Kozak MJ, Foa EB. Obsessions, overvalued ideas, and delusions in obsessive-compulsive disorder. Behav Res Ther. 1994;32(3):343–53. https://doi.org/10.1016/0005-7967(94)90132-5.

Lakhani A, Gandhi K, Collumbien M. Addressing semen loss concerns: towards culturally appropriate HIV/AIDS interventions in Gujarat, India. Reprod Health Matters. 2001;9(18):49–59. https://doi.org/10.1016/S0968-8080(01)90090-4.

Littlewood R. Psychiatry's culture. Int J Soc Psychiatry. 1996;42(4):245–68. https://doi.org/10.1177/002076409604200402.
Madeira L, Leal B, Filipe T, Rodrigues MF, Figueira ML. The uncanny of the illness experience: can phenomenology help? Psychopathology. 2019;52:275–82. https://doi.org/10.1159/000504141.
Maheshwari PN, Tillu ND, Shah US. Extreme self-mutilation due to Dhat syndrome. Indian J Urol. 2022;38(3):243–4. https://doi.org/10.4103/iju.iju_94_22.
Malhotra HK, Wig NN. Dhat syndrome: a culture-bound sex neurosis of the orient. Arch Sex Behav. 1975;4(5):519–28. https://doi.org/10.1007/BF01542130.
Mangot AG, Siddiqui F, Murthy VS. Prevalence and pattern of misconceptions about semen loss and sexual prowess among male medical interns. Med J Dr D Y Patil Vidhyapeeth. 2017;10:536–41. https://doi.org/10.4103/MJDRDYPU.MJDRDYPU_16_17.
Manjula M, Prasadarao PSDV, Kumaraiah V, Mishra H, Raguram R. Sexual dysfunction in single males: a perspective from India. J Clin Psychol. 2003;59(6):701–13. https://doi.org/10.1002/jclp.10153.
Markova IS, Berrios GE. Delusional misidentifications: facts and fancies. Psychopathology. 1994;27(3–5):136–43. https://doi.org/10.1159/000284860.
Matsunaga H, Kiriike N, Matsui T, Iwasaki Y, Stein DJ. Taijin kyofusho: a form of social anxiety disorder that responds to serotonin reuptake inhibitors? Int J Neuropsychopharmacol. 2001;4(3):231–7. https://doi.org/10.1017/s1461145701002474.
McKenna PJ. Disorders with overvalued ideas. Br J Psychiatry. 1984;145:579–85. https://doi.org/10.1192/bjp.145.6.579.
Mehra A, Kathirvel S, Gainder S, Avasthi A, Grover S. Female Dhat syndrome in primary care setting. Ind Psychiatry J. 2021;30:278–84. https://doi.org/10.4103/ipj.ipj_76_20.
Menendez V, Fernandez-Suarez A, Placer J, Garcia-Linares M, Tarragon S, Liso E. Dhat syndrome, an emergent condition within urology in Spain. World J Urol. 2013;31(4):941–5. https://doi.org/10.1007/s00345-012-0911-4.
Mitra S, Singh M, Sinha V, Anwar Z. "Dhat syndrome"—how a man lost his bones! Asian J Psychiatr. 2017;28:181–2. https://doi.org/10.1016/j.ajp.2017.06.004.
Money J, Prakasam KS, Joshi VN. Semen-conservation doctrine from ancient Ayurvedic to modern sexological theory. Am J Psychother. 1991;45(1):9–13. https://doi.org/10.1176/appi.psychotherapy.1991.45.1.9.
Mountjoy RL, Farhall JF, Rossell SL. A phenomenological investigation of overvalued ideas and delusions in clinical and subclinical anorexia nervosa. Psychiatry Res. 2014;220(1-2):507–12. https://doi.org/10.1016/j.psychres.2014.07.073.
Mullen R, Linscott RJ. A comparison of delusions and overvalued ideas. J Nerv Ment Dis. 2010;198(1):35–8. https://doi.org/10.1097/nmd.0b013e3181c818b2.
Mumford DB. The 'Dhat syndrome': a culturally determined symptom of depression? Acta Psychiatr Scand. 1996;94(3):163–7. https://doi.org/10.1111/j.1600-0447.1996.tb09842.x.
Pilowsky I, Spence N, Cobb J, Katsikitis M. The Illness Behavior Questionnaire as an aid to clinical assessment. Gen Hosp Psychiatry. 1984;6:123–30. https://doi.org/10.1016/0163-8343(84)90070-7.
Prakash O. Lessons for postgraduate trainees about Dhat syndrome. Indian J Psychiatry. 2007;49(3):208–10. https://doi.org/10.4103/0019-5545.37324.
Prakash S. The varied presentations of dhat syndrome. World J Urol. 2013;31(4):1015. https://doi.org/10.1007/s00345-012-0992-0.
Prakash S, Mandal P. Is the DSM-5 position on dhat syndrome justified. Asian J Psychiatr. 2014;12:155–7. https://doi.org/10.1016/j.ajp.2014.08.006.
Prakash S, Mandal P. Is Dhat syndrome indeed a culturally determined form of depression? Indian J Psychol Med. 2015;37(1):107–9. https://doi.org/10.4103/0253-7176.150860.
Prakash O, Kar SK, Rao TSS. Indian story on semen loss and related Dhat syndrome. Indian J Psychiatry. 2014;56(4):377–82. https://doi.org/10.4103/0019-5545.146532.
Prakash S, Sharan P, Sood M. A study on phenomenology of Dhat syndrome in men in a general medical setting. Indian J Psychiatry. 2016;58(2):129–41. https://doi.org/10.4103/0019-5545.183776.

Prakash S, Sharan P, Sood M. A qualitative study on psychopathology of dhat syndrome in men: implications for classification of disorders. Asian J Psychiatr. 2018;35:79–88. https://doi.org/10.1016/j.ajp.2018.05.007.

Rajesh G, Jacob KS. Form-content dichotomy in psychopathology. Br J Psychiatry. 2004;185:520–1. https://doi.org/10.1192/bjp.185.6.520-b.

Rajkumar RP, Bharadwaj B. Dhat syndrome: evidence for a depressive spectrum subtype. Asian J Psychiatr. 2014;9:57–60. https://doi.org/10.1016/j.ajp.2014.01.007.

Singh G. Dhat syndrome revisited. Indian J Psychiatry. 1985;27(2):119–22.

Singh G, Avasthi A, Pravin D. Dhat syndrome in a female—a case report. Indian J Psychiatry. 2001;43(4):345–8.

Smith DW. Phenomenology. In: Zalta EN, editor. The Stanford Encyclopedia of Philosophy. 2013, December 16. https://plato.stanford.edu/archives/sum2018/entries/phenomenology/.

Sumathipala A, Siribaddana SH, Bhugra D. Culture-bound syndromes: the story of dhat syndrome. Br J Psychiatry. 2004;184:200–9. https://doi.org/10.1192/bjp.184.3.200.

Telles-Correia D, Sampaio D. Editorial: historical roots of psychopathology. Front Psychol. 2016;7:905. https://doi.org/10.3389/fpsyg.2016.00905.

Tripathi A, Roy D, Kar SK. Distress due to nonpathological vaginal discharge: a new face of Dhat syndrome in females. J Psychosex Health. 2021;3(4):315–21. https://doi.org/10.1177/26318318211049547.

Visser S, Bouman TK. Cognitive-behavioural approaches in the treatment of hypochondriasis: six single case cross-over studies. Behav Res Ther. 1992;30(3):301–6.

Vivekanandan KS, Thangadurai P, Prasad J, Jacob KS. Sexual dysfunction among men in rural Tamil Nadu: nature, prevalence, clinical features, and explanatory models. Indian J Psychol Med. 2019;41(1):81–6. https://doi.org/10.4103/ijpsym.ijpsym_153_18.

War RJ, Albert S. Sexuality and 'silence' among Khasi youth of Meghalaya, Northeast India. Cult Health Sex. 2013;15:S351–64. https://doi.org/10.1080/13691058.2013.792955.

Wig N. Problems of mental health in India. J Clin Soc Psychol (India). 1960;17:48–53.

# Chapter 2
# Epidemiology of Dhat Syndrome

**Swapnajeet Sahoo and Rahul Chakravarty**

## 2.1 Introduction

The concept of culture-bound syndromes refers to psychopathological entities that are geographically defined and largely determined by the beliefs and assumptions of the native culture. The term was first introduced by Yap in the 1950s (Yap 1967). In many cultures, including Indian culture, masculinity is often associated with sexual performance and personal fulfillment, leading to psychological distress related to semen loss (Kulhara and Avasthi 1995). Dhat syndrome is a condition that has been mostly observed in South Asian countries like India, Sri Lanka, and Bangladesh. However, studies have shown that it is also prevalent in other regions outside of South Asia. Literature from various non-South Asian countries such as China, Russia, Europe, and the United States has described Dhat syndrome at different points in time (Avasthi and Jhirwal 2005; Sumathipala et al. 2004).

Dhat syndrome is regarded as the "*neurosis of the orient*" (Malhotra and Wig 1975) but it has shown a global presence, like "*shen-k'uei*" in China (Tan 1980; Wen and Wang 1980). There is evidence from the nineteenth century that similar syndromes were prevalent in Europe, Australia, and the USA. However, these syndromes gradually disappeared due to changes in social and economic factors (Prakash 2007). Semen has been referred to as a "soul substance" by Galen and Aristotle and the physical and psychological symptoms have been attributed to the semen loss (Jadhav 2004). However, many developed countries now have more scientific explanations for bodily/psychic discomfort (Jadhav 2007). Distress has not disappeared in developed countries, but now manifests as psychological and somatic symptoms (Balhara 2011). Despite adequate evidence about the existence of Dhat syndrome, it has not yet been considered as a distinct identity in the *Diagnostic and Statistical Manual of Mental Disorders* (DSM-5) (*Diagnostic and Statistical*

S. Sahoo (✉) · R. Chakravarty
Department of Psychiatry, PGIMER, Chandigarh, India

© The Author(s), under exclusive license to Springer Nature Singapore Pte Ltd. 2024

S. K. Kar et al. (eds.), *Dhat Syndrome*,
https://doi.org/10.1007/978-981-99-8870-9_2

*Manual of Mental Disorders* 2013) or in the recent 11th edition of the *International Classification of Diseases* (ICD-11) (World Health Organization 2022, p. 11).

Being a culture-bound syndrome, the epidemiology of Dhat syndrome can vary within different populations and cultural contexts. Nonetheless, several studies have explored the phenomenon to better understand its prevalence and associated factors. The prevalence of Dhat syndrome varies across studies, ranging from 4 to 58% among male patients seeking treatment for sexual disorders in South Asian clinical settings (Strong et al. 2022). The wide range suggests that diagnostic criteria employed and cultural factors in different studies may contribute to the variation (Alarcón 2009).

## 2.2 Frequency

Studies have reported Dhat syndrome to be present in 64.6–76.7% of male patients with psychosexual disorders, that results in its recognition as the most common culture-bound syndrome in the Indian subcontinent (Bhatia 1999; Bhatia and Malik 1991; Rao 2021). A systematic review of 13 studies involving male patients suffering from Dhat syndrome reported the mean age of the patients to be 26 years (Udina et al. 2013). In this study, the patients described Dhat syndrome as having a fear of semen loss. Out of these 13 studies, 11 were from India, one was from Sri Lanka and one from Europe (Udina et al. 2013). However, this systematic review only analysed studies which had only male patients and did not mention the existence of Dhat syndrome in females (Udina et al. 2013).

During a recent study, 70 healthcare professionals working in outpatient clinics were approached to collect demographic data on 1777 male patients with Dhat syndrome. The patients' ages ranged from 12 to 65 years old. Results showed that the majority of patients had a low socioeconomic status, lower educational attainment in comparison to their peers, and were living without spouse (Khan 2005). Sociodemography of first-time patients of a referred psychosexual clinic in North India also revealed similar findings and also found that the majority of patients followed Hinduism, and hailed from rural locations (Grover et al. 2016b).

## 2.3 Distribution

Most mental health professionals think that Dhat syndrome is limited to the Indian subcontinent, but the reports of its existence have been described outside of the Indian subcontinent as well and hence, can be said to be a global phenomenon (Deb and Balhara 2013). A study from urological services in Spain from 2006–2007 described 32 patients having symptoms consistent with Dhat syndrome (Menéndez et al. 2013). These patients were immigrants from South Asian regions. The authors stressed the importance of quickly identifying this syndrome to improve the quality of care. This includes reducing unnecessary testing, especially since Spanish healthcare providers have limited knowledge of Dhat syndrome and there are increasing numbers of immigrants (Menéndez et al. 2013). A study on a Muslim patient in Oman found that cultural beliefs shared by both Muslim and Indian communities, which prohibit activities that lead to semen release, may be a contributing factor to Dhat syndrome. This suggests that Dhat syndrome may be a response to cultural inhibitions rather than a syndrome specific to a particular culture (MacFarland et al. 2017). Similarly, in the United Kingdom, 47 white patients were found to experience Dhat-like symptomology by a psychiatrist of South Asian descent (Jadhav 2007). Perhaps the health care providers are often not familiar with such syndromes and label them as some specific type of phobia or anxiety (Strong et al. 2022).

## 2.4 Determinants

### *2.4.1 Gender*

Male patients who exhibit symptoms of Dhat syndrome are typically individuals who have recently gotten married, belong to lower or middle socio-economic backgrounds (such as students, laborers, or farmers), come from rural areas, and are usually from families with conservative views regarding sexual matters (Behere and Natraj 1984; Bhatia and Malik 1991; Chadda and Ahuja 1990). The cause and symptoms of Dhat syndrome are linked to cultural beliefs about the negative effects of semen loss on health (Strong et al. 2022). Beliefs surrounding the importance of semen and its loss during certain activities, such as masturbation or nocturnal emissions, are cultural factors that significantly contribute to the development and continuation of Dhat syndrome. Those with this syndrome often experience a variety of psychological symptoms, including depression, physical complaints, anxiety, exhaustion, and sexual dysfunction (typically erectile dysfunction). Many patients attribute their excessive masturbation as the primary cause of their distress, as they believe it results in an ongoing loss of semen through urine (Rao 2021). These symptoms, physical and psychological, can greatly impact quality of life and functioning and sometimes result in disability (Shahi et al. 2022).

It has been documented that there is a female version of Dhat syndrome which shares some similarities with the male version but also has distinct differences. Studies have found that the average age of onset for females with Dhat syndrome is higher than that of males, with females experiencing symptoms at around 36.1 years of age compared to 24 years for males (Mehra et al. 2021). In female Dhat syndrome, the reasons given by patients differ from those of males. A study conducted by Mehra et al. involved 69 females with nonpathological vaginal discharge that was consistent with female Dhat syndrome. These women did not show any signs of infection, and the amount of discharge was similar to normal physiological conditions. The most common attribution to the reported discharge was the consumption of warm foods and drinks (75.8%), followed by eating unbalanced or inappropriate food (73.5%) (Mehra et al. 2021). The reasons behind these reactions could be related to traditional Indian Aryuvedic medicine. According to ancient Aryuvedic textbooks, it is advisable to avoid certain foods like ghee, eggs, or meat because they generate excess humoral heat. Females who suffer from Dhat syndrome associate their symptoms with the discharge of Dhat and experience somatic symptoms similar to their male counterparts. Some women also experience weakness and bodily concerns due to wetness during sexual intercourse, which is similar to male Dhat syndrome. A majority of these patients believe that their vaginal discharge is responsible for bodily weakness (87%), backache (71%), and stomach-ache (66.7%) (Mehra et al. 2021). This is because they believe that they are losing a vital fluid of the body, which they refer to as "safed paani" or white water in Hindi, which is similar to Dhat in males. Studies have primarily focused on female Dhat syndrome(Grover et al. 2014, 2016a), still, there is much to be understood and explored about this condition. The criteria for diagnosing female Dhat syndrome is unclear, especially because normal vaginal discharge can be a sign of sexual communication, social distress or psychological problems.

### *2.4.2 Socio-demographic Factors in Dhat Syndrome*

It has been suggested that certain socio-demographic factors, including nuptiality, income, and educational attainment, may be associated with Dhat syndrome. However, research findings on this topic are mixed. Some studies indicate that the condition is more common among unmarried individuals with lower incomes and levels of education, while other variables such as age and place of origin may also play a role. In a study with a large sample size of 269 patients with Dhat syndrome, the condition was found to be more common in rural areas and families with conservative attitudes towards sexuality. Factors such as place of origin, irregular salary, and never-married status were also associated with the condition (Deb and Balhara 2013). Although Dhat syndrome has its cultural origins, it is also linked to specific medical interpretations. Certain people may seek medical assistance for physical symptoms like fatigue, weakness, and urinary issues that they attribute to semen loss. However, medical assessments usually do not detect any physiological abnormalities.

## 2.5 Symptomatology

Patients, in addition to experiencing sexual complaints also report various psychosomatic symptoms. Studies have shown that those with Dhat syndrome may experience bodily weakness, mental weakness, pain in various parts of the body, decreased interest in pleasurable activities, fatigue, depressed mood, poor concentration, and anger episodes. These symptoms were present in more than half of the study population (Deb and Balhara 2013; Dhungana et al. 2017; Gautham et al. 2008; Grover et al. 2015) (Table 2.1).

Some studies categorised the symptoms into four categories, namely, somatic symptoms, anxiety symptoms, depressive symptoms, and sexual symptoms (Balhara 2011; Bhatia 1999; Bhatia and Malik 1991; Chadda and Ahuja 1990; Deb and Balhara 2013; Jadhav 2004) (Table 2.2).

Various studies (Avasthi et al. 2012; Bhatti and Fikree 2002; Grover et al. 2014; Patel et al. 2005, 2008; Singh et al. 2001; Trollope-Kumar 2001) have tried to compare the symptomatology of male dhat syndrome with female dhat syndrome. They found that demographic factors, clinical factors and psychosomatic symptoms were comparable in both populations. In sexual symptoms, males reported premature ejaculation and erectile dysfunction as major symptoms, while females reported sexual weakness and lack of desire as major sexual symptoms (Table 2.3).

**Table 2.1** Symptoms in patients of Dhat Syndromes (Deb and Balhara 2013; Dhungana et al. 2017; Gautham et al. 2008; Grover et al. 2015)

| Complaints | Prevalence (%) |
|---|---|
| Bodily weakness | 78–80 |
| Mental weakness | 62–76 |
| Back pain | 46–52 |
| Pain in extremities, or joints (knees, hips, etc.) | 51–58 |
| Dizziness | 39–48 |
| Feeling your heart pound or race | 38–40 |
| Constipation, loose bowels, or diarrhoea | 18–32 |
| Nausea, gas or indigestion | 32–40 |
| Little interest or pleasure in doing things | 63–80 |
| Feeling tired or having low energy | 67–76 |
| Feeling down, depressed or hopeless | 62–74 |
| Anorexia or overeating | 24–48 |
| Feeling bad about yourself that you are a failure | 32–50 |
| Burning micturition | 42–52 |
| Trouble concentrating on things | 49–62 |
| Difficulty in gaining weight or losing weight | 24–38 |
| Excessive worry | 56–96 |
| Anger, irritability, getting annoyed easily | 48–56 |

**Table 2.2** Summary of presenting symptoms by patients with Dhat syndrome (Balhara 2011; Bhatia 1999; Bhatia and Malik 1991; Chadda and Ahuja 1990; Deb and Balhara 2013; Jadhav 2004)

| Somatic symptoms | Anxiety symptoms | Depressive symptoms | Sexual symptoms |
|---|---|---|---|
| • Multiple body aches<br>• Burning micturition<br>• Increased frequency of micturition<br>• Difficulty in micturition<br>• Hollowing of eyes<br>• Loss of control over the body<br>• Loss of control over the mind<br>• Vertigo<br>• Swelling of the body<br>• Distension of abdomen<br>• Belching<br>• Gas formation<br>• Epigastric pain<br>• Lumbar pain<br>• Involuntary passage of stool during micturition | • Anxiety<br>• Dryness of mouth/ throat<br>• Palpitation<br>• Tachycardia<br>• Increased muscle tension<br>• Fear of losing vital components of the body | • Weakness<br>• Guilt<br>• Lethargy<br>• Loss of appetite<br>• Sleep disturbance<br>• Loss of interest<br>• Loss of attention/ concentration<br>• Loss of memory<br>• Weight loss<br>• Suicidal ideation<br>• Feeling of shame | • Distortion of the shape of the penis<br>• Genital itching<br>• Genital boils and ulcers<br>• Fear of sexual activity<br>• Loss of libido<br>• Erectile dysfunction<br>• Premature ejaculation<br>• Impotence |

**Table 2.3** Comparison of symptomatology of male and female Dhat Syndrome (Avasthi et al. 2012; Bhatti and Fikree 2002; Grover et al. 2014; Patel et al. 2005, 2008; Singh et al. 2001; Trollope-Kumar 2001)

| Clinical factors | Dhat syndrome in males | Dhat syndrome in females |
|---|---|---|
| Age group | Young | Young |
| Educational status | Lower educational | Illiterate or low education |
| Marital status | Recently married | Recently married |
| Locality | Rural | Rural |
| Characteristics of discharge | Usually whitish and odourless | whitish and odourless |
| Local physical examination | No evidence of infection | No or little evidence of infection |
| Laboratory examination | No evidence of semen or infection | No evidence of infection |
| Physical symptoms | Fatigue, lethargy, loss of appetite, lack of physical strength | Burning of hands and feet, dizziness, backache and weakness |
| Mental state | Worried/preoccupied with the loss of precious and vital body secretion | Worried about loss of genital secretions |
| Mental symptoms | Poor concentration, forgetfulness, anxiety and depressive symptoms | Poor concentration, anxiety and depressive symptoms |
| Sexual dysfunction | Premature ejaculation or erectile dysfunction | Sexual weakness, loss of libido |
| Psychiatric morbidity | Depressive disorder or generalized anxiety disorder | Depression |

## 2.6 Conclusions and Future Directions

Dhat syndrome is a complex clinical condition that is unique to certain cultures and can be a topic of fascination and controversy. It encompasses a range of physical and mental symptoms that may also be present in populations beyond the Indian sub-continent. Strong correlations have been found between Dhat syndrome and sexual and psychiatric disorders, which may stem from distress related to loss of semen. Interestingly, the symptoms of Dhat syndrome are similar between genders and are primarily prevalent in rural populations with lower socio-economic and educational status. As such, effective treatment should prioritize addressing the misconceptions and false beliefs surrounding this condition.

## References

Alarcón RD. Culture, cultural factors and psychiatric diagnosis: review and projections. World Psychiatry. 2009;8(3):131–9.

Avasthi A, Jhirwal O. The concept and epidemiology of Dhat syndrome. J Pak Psychiatr Soc. 2005;2:6–8.

Avasthi A, Grover S, Prakash O. Dhat Syndrome: a culture-bound sex related disorder in Indian subcontinent. In: Sexually transmitted infections. 2nd ed. Elsevier; 2012. p. 1225–30.

Balhara YPS. Culture-bound Syndrome: has it found its right niche? Indian J Psychol Med. 2011;33(2):210–5. https://doi.org/10.4103/0253-7176.92055.

Behere PB, Natraj GS. Dhat Syndrome: the phenomenology of a culture bound sex neurosis of the orient. Indian J Psychiatry. 1984;26(1):76–8.

Bhatia MS. An analysis of 60 cases of culture bound syndromes. Indian J Med Sci. 1999;53(4):149–52.

Bhatia MS, Malik SC. Dhat syndrome—a useful diagnostic entity in Indian culture. Br J Psychiatry J Ment Sci. 1991;159:691–5. https://doi.org/10.1192/bjp.159.5.691.

Bhatti LI, Fikree FF. Health-seeking behavior of Karachi women with reproductive tract infections. Social Science & Medicine (1982). 2002;54(1):105–17. https://doi.org/10.1016/s0277-9536(01)00012-0.

Chadda RK, Ahuja N. Dhat syndrome. A sex neurosis of the Indian subcontinent. Br J Psychiatry J Ment Sci. 1990;156:577–9. https://doi.org/10.1192/bjp.156.4.577.

Deb KS, Balhara YPS. Dhat syndrome: a review of the world literature. Indian J Psychol Med. 2013;35(4):326–31. https://doi.org/10.4103/0253-7176.122219.

Dhungana M, Ghimire SR, Thapa M. A study of Dhat syndrome—a culture bound syndrome in Nepalese context. J Psychiatr Assoc Nepal. 2017;6(1) https://doi.org/10.3126/jpan.v6i1.21770. Article 1.

Diagnostic and statistical manual of mental disorders: DSM-5™. 5th ed. American Psychiatric Publishing, Inc.; 2013. pp. xliv, 947. https://doi.org/10.1176/appi.books.9780890425596.

Gautham M, Singh R, Weiss H, Brugha R, Patel V, Desai NG, Nandan D, Kielmann K, Grosskurth H. Socio-cultural, psychosexual and biomedical factors associated with genital symptoms experienced by men in rural India. Trop Med Int Health. 2008;13(3):384–95. https://doi.org/10.1111/j.1365-3156.2008.02013.x.

Grover S, Kate N, Avasthi A, Rajpal N, Umamaheswari V. Females too suffer from Dhat syndrome: a case series and revisit of the concept. Indian J Psychiatry. 2014;56(4):388–92. https://doi.org/10.4103/0019-5545.146537.

Grover S, Avasthi A, Gupta S, Dan A, Neogi R, Behere PB, Lakdawala B, Tripathi A, Chakraborty K, Sinha V, Bhatia MS, Pattojoshi A, Rao TSS, Rozatkar A. Comorbidity in patients with Dhat syndrome: a nationwide multicentric study. J Sex Med. 2015;12(6):1398–401. https://doi.org/10.1111/jsm.12899.

Grover S, Avasthi A, Gupta S, Hazari N, Malhotra N. Do female patients with nonpathological vaginal discharge need the same evaluation as for Dhat syndrome in males? Indian J Psychiatry. 2016a;58(1):61–9. https://doi.org/10.4103/0019-5545.174376.

Grover S, Gupta S, Avasthi A. A follow-up study of patients with Dhat syndrome: treatment pattern, outcome, and reasons for dropout from treatment. Indian J Psychiatry. 2016b;58(1):49–56. https://doi.org/10.4103/0019-5545.174373.

Jadhav S. Dhāt syndrome: a re-evaluation. Psychiatry. 2004;3(8):14–6. https://doi.org/10.1383/psyt.3.8.14.43399.

Jadhav S. Dhis and Dhāt: evidence of semen retention syndrome amongst white Britons. Anthropol Med. 2007;14(3):229–39. https://doi.org/10.1080/13648470701772770.

Khan N. Dhat syndrome in relation to demographic characteristics. Indian J Psychiatry. 2005;47(1):54–7. https://doi.org/10.4103/0019-5545.46077.

Kulhara P, Avasthi A. Sexual dysfunction on the indian subcontinent. Int Rev Psychiatry. 1995;7(2):231–9. https://doi.org/10.3109/09540269509028331.

MacFarland AS, Al-Maashani M, Al Busaidi Q, Al-Naamani A, El-Bouri M, Al-Adawi S. Culture-specific pathogenicity of Dhat (semen loss) syndrome in an Arab/Islamic Society, Oman. Oman Med J. 2017;32(3):251–5. https://doi.org/10.5001/omj.2017.47.

Malhotra HK, Wig NN. Dhat syndrome: a culture-bound sex neurosis of the orient. Arch Sex Behav. 1975;4(5):519–28. https://doi.org/10.1007/BF01542130.

Mehra A, Kathirvel S, Gainder S, Avasthi A, Grover S. Female Dhat syndrome in primary care setting. Ind Psychiatry J. 2021;30(2):278–84. https://doi.org/10.4103/ipj.ipj_76_20.

Menéndez V, Fernández-Suárez A, Placer J, García-Linares M, Tarragon S, Liso E. Dhat syndrome, an emergent condition within urology in Spain. World J Urol. 2013;31(4):941–5. https://doi.org/10.1007/s00345-012-0911-4.

Patel V, Pednekar S, Weiss H, Rodrigues M, Barros P, Nayak B, Tanksale V, West B, Nevrekar P, Kirkwood BR, Mabey D. Why do women complain of vaginal discharge? A population survey of infectious and pyschosocial risk factors in a South Asian community. Int J Epidemiol. 2005;34(4):853–62. https://doi.org/10.1093/ije/dyi072.

Patel V, Andrew G, Pelto PJ. The psychological and social contexts of complaints of abnormal vaginal discharge: a study of illness narratives in India. J Psychosom Res. 2008;64(3):255–62; discussion 263–4. https://doi.org/10.1016/j.jpsychores.2007.10.015.

Prakash O. Lessons for postgraduate trainees about Dhat syndrome. Indian J Psychiatry. 2007;49(3):208–10. https://doi.org/10.4103/0019-5545.37324.

Rao TSS. History and mystery of Dhat syndrome: a critical look at the current understanding and future directions. Indian J Psychiatry. 2021;63(4):317–25. https://doi.org/10.4103/psychiatry.IndianJPsychiatry_791_20.

Shahi MK, Tripathi A, Singh A, Kar SK, Nischal A, Singh S, Dalal PK. Quality of life and disability in patients with dhat syndrome: a cross-sectional study. Indian J Psychol Med. 2022;44(5):459–65. https://doi.org/10.1177/02537176221078422.

Singh G, Avasthi A, Pravin D. Dhat syndrome in a female—a case report. Indian J Psychiatry. 2001;43(4):345–8.

Strong YN, Li A, White ME, Razzak AN, Anderson DJ, Kaye AD, Herron EW, Khater NP, Bradley EC, Urits I. Dhat Syndrome: epidemiology, risk factors, comorbidities, diagnosis, treatment, and management. Health Psychol Res. 2022;10(4):38759. https://doi.org/10.52965/001c.38759.

Sumathipala A, Siribaddana SH, Bhugra D. Culture-bound syndromes: the story of dhat syndrome. Br J Psychiatry J Ment Sci. 2004;184:200–9. https://doi.org/10.1192/bjp.184.3.200.

Tan E. Culture-bound syndromes among overseas Chinese. In: Normal and abnormal lbehavior in Chinese culture. Dordrecht: D Reidel Publishing Co.; 1980. p. 371–86.

Trollope-Kumar K. Cultural and biomedical meanings of the complaint of leukorrhea in South Asian women. Trop Med Int Health. 2001;6(4):260–6. https://doi.org/10.1046/j.1365-3156.2001.00699.x.

Udina M, Foulon H, Valdés M, Bhattacharyya S, Martín-Santos R. Dhat syndrome: a systematic review. Psychosomatics. 2013;54(3):212–8. https://doi.org/10.1016/j.psym.2012.09.003.

Wen J, Wang C. Shen-kui syndrome: a culture-specific sexual neurosis in Taiwan. In: Normal and abnormal behaviour in Chinese culture. Dordrecht: D Reidel Publishing Co.; 1980. p. 357–69.

World Health Organization. ICD-11. 2022. https://icd.who.int/en.

Yap PM. Classification of the culture-bound reactive syndromes. Aust N Z J Psychiatry. 1967;1(4):172–9. https://doi.org/10.3109/00048676709159191.

# Chapter 3
# Dhat Syndrome as a Diagnostic Category: The Nosological Struggle

**Sujita Kumar Kar, Vikas Menon, and S. M. Yasir Arafat**

## 3.1 Introduction

Dhat syndrome is a well-recognized culture-bound syndrome commonly seen in young, unmarried, less educated males from rural backgrounds in South East Asia (Kar et al. 2021a). It is also popularly known by the names "Semen loss anxiety" and "semen loss syndrome" (Kar et al. 2021a). Dhat syndrome is commonly presently with anxiety, depression, and somatic symptoms, where the whole attribution of the symptoms goes to semen loss by any means (Bhatia and Malik 1991; Deb and Balhara 2013; Kar and Sarkar 2015; Prakash and Kar 2019). Myths related to sexuality are the major cause of erratic attribution of the symptoms of semen loss. Dhat syndrome significantly affects the quality of life and also significantly disabling (Shahi et al. 2022). There is significant variations in the phenomenology of the symptoms of dhat syndrome among the patients and the comorbidities also vary between the patients needing a person-centred management (Kar and Singh 2016). A similar entity is also prevalent in females, where females attribute anxiety, depression and somatic complaints to non-pathological vaginal discharge (Chaturvedi et al. 1993). It is commonly called female dhat syndrome and it produces significant distress and disability in the patients (Joshi et al. 2022). Despite being commonly encountered in clinical practice, many of these patients were diagnosed with somatoform disorder, anxiety disorder, depression or sexual dysfunctions due to the phenomenological similarity between these conditions (Kar and Sarkar 2015). The

S. K. Kar (✉)
Department of Psychiatry, King George's Medical University, Lucknow, Uttar Pradesh, India

V. Menon
Department of Psychiatry, Jawaharlal Institute of Postgraduate Medical Education and Research (JIPMER), Puducherry, Tamil Nadu, India

S. M. Y. Arafat
Department of Psychiatry, Enam Medical College and Hospital, Dhaka, Bangladesh

© The Author(s), under exclusive license to Springer Nature Singapore Pte Ltd. 2024
S. K. Kar et al. (eds.), *Dhat Syndrome*,
https://doi.org/10.1007/978-981-99-8870-9_3

diagnosis of Dhat syndrome in females faces similar challenges (Kar and Singh 2017). The diagnostic stability of Dhat syndrome is also questioned in research (Sameer et al. 2015; Sridhar et al. 2018). This chapter will discuss nosological status and dilemmas in the diagnosis of Dhat syndrome.

## 3.2 The Birth of Dhat Syndrome

A pioneer of Indian psychiatry Prof. N. N. Wig first used the term "Dhat syndrome" and defined this entity as an important diagnostic entity in the 1960s (Kar and Mishra 2018; Wig 1960). Subsequently, researchers emphasized the importance of this entity in their research (Behere and Natraj 1984; Bhatia and Malik 1991; Chadda and Ahuja 1990; Malhotra and Wig 1975). Dhat syndrome was described as "Culture bound sex neurosis of the Orient" (Behere and Natraj 1984; Malhotra and Wig 1975) and "Sex neurosis of the Indian subcontinent" (Chadda and Ahuja 1990). As a significant number of patients were consulting the psychiatric clinics with concerns related to loss of semen and feared some dreadful consequences of it, it was considered as useful clinical diagnostic entity (Bhatia et al. 1989; Bhatia and Malik 1991). Patients with Dhat syndrome often harbour a strong belief about the preciousness of semen and the serious consequences associated with semen loss, which are often linked to ancient culture-religious beliefs (Kar and Sarkar 2015; Prakash et al. 2014). All the religious texts globally emphasize the preservation of semen for longevity and a healthy life (Prakash et al. 2014; Sumathipala et al. 2004). Though this entity was labelled as dhat syndrome by Prof. Wig in the 1960s, it is existing since ancient times and might have a different name across the regions, globally. This entity (which is now known as dhat syndrome) is being treated as an illness since ancient times by traditional and religious healers. Over the past six decades several research works were done on dhat syndrome and most of the research are done in South East Asia (particularly India) by psychiatrists (Kar et al. 2021b). Most research on dhat syndrome occurred during the past decade. Research on Dhat syndrome mostly focuses on phenomenology, sociocultural aspects, comorbidities associated, nosological status and management for Dhat syndrome (Kar et al. 2021b).

## 3.3 Dhat Syndrome in International Classificatory System

Dhat syndrome started its journey as a separate identity in the 1960s in India. However, during the last more than half a century, it is yet to have a definitive position in international classificatory systems (Arafat 2017). It was first included in the International Classificatory Systems, i.e. in the *International Classification of Diseases* (ICD) version 10 and for the first time Dhat syndrome got a place as a diagnosis entity, in the ICD-10 and the *Diagnostic and Statistical Manual of Mental*

*Disorders* (DSM), Text Revision of the fourth edition (DSM-IV-TR) (Sridhar et al. 2018; World Health Organization 1994; American Psychiatric Association 2000). The DSM-IV TR had included DS under the section "Glossary of culture-bound syndromes" and described it as a 'folk diagnostic term' associated with marked anxiety and hypochondriacal concerns about loss of semen. In DSM-5, DS is now placed under the section "Glossary of cultural concepts of distress". It clarifies that DS, despite its name, is not a separate syndrome but a culturally favoured explanation of distress related to loss of *dhat* without any identifiable physiological dysfunction (American Psychiatric Association 2013; Arafat 2017). In the ICD, the change in the nosological status of Dhat syndrome has been even more striking. Whereas in ICD-10, DS enjoyed the status of a separate diagnostic entity under the category of "other specified neurotic disorders", it does not find a mention in ICD-11 (World Health Organization 2022; Sharan and Hans 2021).

## 3.4 Dhat Syndrome Diagnosis: Controversies

The nosological status of Dhat syndrome (DS) has been an enduring controversy. Despite its cultural significance and widespread acceptance in South Asian cultures, several factors contribute to the controversies surrounding the nosological status of DS:

### *3.4.1 Cultural Boundaries (Is It Culture Bound?)*

DS has traditionally been described as a 'neurosis of the Orient' and viewed as a 'culture-bound syndrome (CBS)'. However, researchers have cautioned that categorizing CBS separately, by itself, does not improve the recognition or management of these conditions (Wig 1994). Littlewood (1996) has argued for dropping the concept of CBS because all psychiatric syndromes are inherently culture-bound and because these syndromes lack distinct phenomenological and epidemiological patterns (Littlewood, 1996). Further, with increasing globalization, these syndromes are likely to become less apparent. Some critics argue that its inclusion in mainstream diagnostic systems may perpetuate cultural stereotypes and medicalize cultural norms. On the other hand, it has been identified outside the Indian subcontinent namely China, Malaysia, Japan, USA, Russia, Spain, and countries in central Asia. This distribution can be attributed to the migration of South Asian populations there. Along with these distributions, the importance of semen was also described in the writings of Galen, Aristotle, Beard, Hare, and Maudsley where semen loss was attributed to psychiatric illness (Arafat 2017).

### 3.4.2 Overlapping Symptoms (Is It a Symptom of Depression?)

Phenomenologically, DS has significant overlap with anxiety, somatoform, and depressive disorders. As an example, symptoms of fatigue, lassitude, palpitations, and insomnia seen in DS can overlap with anxiety and depression. This overlap in symptoms has led researchers to question the merits of a separate diagnostic status for Dhat syndrome. In a retrospective investigation, Rajkumar and Bharadwaj (2014) showed that a subset of people with DS may be better viewed as having a depressive spectrum disorder with higher rates of depressive symptoms and a positive family history of depression. This extended the findings of Mumford (1996), two decades earlier, who concluded that depression is a culturally sanctioned manifestation of depression (Mumford, 1996). An alternate conceptualization may be that DS is merely a cultural concept or idiom of distress. It is possible that depressive cognitions may underlie the attributional errors seen in DS and this attitude is subsequently maintained by an interplay of cultural attitudes towards sexuality and learned helplessness (Rao 2021).

### 3.4.3 Lack of Objective Markers or Specific Criteria (Is It Non-specific?)

Unlike many medical conditions with identifiable biomarkers, DS lacks definitive biological evidence. The diagnosis primarily relies on a combination of self-reported symptoms, cultural beliefs surrounding the origin of symptoms (loss of semen), and resultant psychological distress, making it challenging to establish clear diagnostic criteria. Indeed, Balhara (2011) has argued that the emotional distress and cultural context underlying DS are not specific and can be seen in other psychiatric disorders.

### 3.4.4 Evolving Cultural Perceptions (Is It Temporary?)

As societies undergo rapid modernization and cultural shifts, the prevalence and significance of DS may change accordingly. What was once a widely recognized and significant syndrome in a specific cultural context might gradually lose its prominence. This may make it difficult to frame enduring diagnostic criteria for DS. Recognizing cultural dynamics and adopting a culturally sensitive approach is essential in addressing the controversies surrounding the nosological status of Dhat syndrome. However, it is important to consider that, the epidemiology of any disorder may change over time. And secondly, since the 1960s, it has been persistent in Indian Sub-continent.

### *3.4.5 Alternative Explanations (Is It Somatization?)*

DS is deeply rooted in cultural beliefs about semen and its significance. In societies where the syndrome is prevalent, semen is often regarded as a vital life force, and its loss is believed to lead to physical and mental health problems. The alternative perspective acknowledges that these cultural beliefs play a crucial role in shaping how individuals perceive and interpret their symptoms. The distress experienced by DS sufferers may be moderated by underlying sexual anxiety and social and psychological pressures related to expectations surrounding masculinity, sexual performance, and reproductive vigour. Other alternate explanations of DS relate to the somatization of psychological distress. There also exists a possibility that DS may have equivalent presentations in different settings and contexts arguing against a one-size-fits-all categorical approach to diagnosis and management.

## 3.5 Future Directions and Conclusion

Dhat syndrome was seen as a prodrome of psychosis(Kar et al. 2017). It was also found to be associated with recurrent brief depressive disorder (Kar and Garg 2016). These associations indicate a strong biological underpinning behind dhat syndrome, rather than it being a purely psycho-socio-cultural syndrome (Kar et al. 2017; Kar and Garg 2016). Accumulating evidence indicates a possible biological basis of Dhat syndrome and future research in a larger population may be able to give better insight to the pathophysiology of Dhat syndrome, which may help in giving recognition to Dhat syndrome in the nosological system and may help in understanding dhat syndrome beyond the cultural boundary. Global acculturation and deculturation, increasing educational level and more migration may affect the cross-cultural presentation of Dhat syndrome (Kar 2015). The manifestation of dhat syndrome in multiple cultures across the globe may affect its cultural identity and culture boundness, making it a non-culture bound psycho-somatic syndrome. Extensive research about this entity across the cultures may give more clarity to this diagnostic entity.

## References

American Psychiatric Association. Diagnostic and statistical manual of mental disorders. 4th ed. Text version. Washington, DC: American Psychiatric Association; 2000.

American Psychiatric Association. Diagnostic and statistical manual of mental disorders. 5th ed. Washington, DC: American Psychiatric Association; 2013.

Arafat SY. Dhat syndrome: culture bound, separate entity, or removed. J Behav Health. 2017;6(3):147–50. https://doi.org/10.5455/jbh.20170123102726.

Balhara YP. Culture-bound Syndrome: has it found its right niche? Indian J Psychol Med. 2011;33(2):210–5. https://doi.org/10.4103/0253-7176.92055.

Behere PB, Natraj GS. Dhat syndrome: the phenomenology of a culture bound sex neurosis of the orient. Indian J Psychiatry. 1984;26(1):76–8.
Bhatia MS, Malik SC. Dhat syndrome—a useful diagnostic entity in Indian culture. Br J Psychiatry J Ment Sci. 1991;159:691–5. https://doi.org/10.1192/bjp.159.5.691.
Bhatia MS, Bohra N, Malik SC. "Dhat" syndrome—a useful clinical entity. Indian J Dermatol. 1989;34(2):32–41.
Chadda RK, Ahuja N. Dhat syndrome. A sex neurosis of the Indian subcontinent. Br J Psychiatry J Ment Sci. 1990;156:577–9. https://doi.org/10.1192/bjp.156.4.577.
Chaturvedi SK, Chandra PS, Isaac MK, Sudarshan CY, Rao S. Is there a female Dhat syndrome. NIMHANS J. 1993;11(2):89–93.
Deb KS, Balhara YPS. Dhat syndrome: a review of the world literature. Indian J Psychol Med. 2013;35(4):326–31. https://doi.org/10.4103/0253-7176.122219.
Joshi S, Tripathi A, Agarwal S, Singh N, Gupta B, Nischal A, Kar SK. Phenomenology, disability and sexual functioning in female Dhat syndrome: a study of tertiary care gynaecology outpatients. Gen Psychiatr. 2022;35(5):e100863. https://doi.org/10.1136/gpsych-2022-100863.
Kar SK. Dhat syndrome: will it reach a height or die soon? J Hum Reprod Sci. 2015;8(4):246. https://doi.org/10.4103/0974-1208.170421.
Kar SK, Garg K. Recurrent brief depressive disorder in Dhat syndrome: a biological or psychological phenomenon! Aust N Z J Psychiatry. 2016;50(3):291–2. https://doi.org/10.1177/0004867415604368.
Kar SK, Mishra SR. Prof. NN Wig & his contribution to understand Dhat syndrome. Indian J Health Sex Cult. 2018;4(2):39–40.
Kar SK, Sarkar S. Dhat syndrome: evolution of concept, current understanding, and need of an integrated approach. J Hum Reprod Sci. 2015;8(3):130–4. https://doi.org/10.4103/0974-1208.165143.
Kar SK, Singh A. Person centered management approach for the Dhat syndrome. Int J Pers Cent Med. 2016;6(4):Article 4. https://doi.org/10.5750/ijpcm.v6i4.615.
Kar SK, Singh A. Where lies the fault in diagnosing Dhat syndrome among females? Understanding through a case study. Indian J Psychol Med. 2017;39(4):506–8. https://doi.org/10.4103/0253-7176.211742.
Kar SK, Shahi MK, Tripathi A. Dhat syndrome as the prodrome of schizophrenia: understanding the cultural distress. Asian J Psychiatr. 2017;25:203–4. https://doi.org/10.1016/j.ajp.2016.11.006.
Kar SK, Arafat SMY, Menon V. A bibliometric analysis of Dhat syndrome. Psychiatry Int. 2021a;2(4):379–85. https://www.mdpi.com/1319004.
Kar SK, Menon V, Arafat SY, Singh A, Das A, Shankar A, Sharma P, Perera S. Dhat syndrome: systematic review of epidemiology, nosology, clinical features, and management strategies. Asian J Psychiatr. 2021b;65:102863. https://doi.org/10.1016/j.ajp.2021.102863.
Littlewood R. Psychiatry's Culture. International Journal of Social Psychiatry. 1996;42(4):245–268. https://doi.org/10.1177/002076409604200402.
Malhotra HK, Wig NN. Dhat syndrome: a culture-bound sex neurosis of the orient. Arch Sex Behav. 1975;4(5):519–28. https://doi.org/10.1007/BF01542130.
Mumford DB. The 'Dhat syndrome': a culturally determined symptom of depression? Acta Psychiatr Scand. 1996;94(3):163–7. https://doi.org/10.1111/j.1600-0447.1996.tb09842.x. PMID: 8891081.
Prakash O, Kar SK. Dhat syndrome: a review and update. J Psychosex Health. 2019. https://doi.org/10.1177/2631831819894769.
Prakash O, Kar SK, Sathyanarayana Rao TS. Indian story on semen loss and related Dhat syndrome. Indian J Psychiatry. 2014;56(4):377–82. https://doi.org/10.4103/0019-5545.146532.
Rajkumar RP, Bharadwaj B. Dhat syndrome: evidence for a depressive spectrum subtype. Asian J Psychiatr. 2014;9:57–60. https://doi.org/10.1016/j.ajp.2014.01.007.
Rao TSS. History and mystery of Dhat syndrome: A critical look at the current understanding and future directions. Indian J Psychiatry. 2021;63(4):317–325. https://doi.org/10.4103/psychiatry.IndianJPsychiatry_791_20.

Sameer M, Menon V, Chandrasekaran R. Is "pure" Dhat syndrome a stable diagnostic entity? A naturalistic long term follow up study from a tertiary care centre. J Clin Diagn Res. 2015;9(8):VC01–3. https://doi.org/10.7860/JCDR/2015/13399.6275.
Shahi MK, Tripathi A, Singh A, Kar SK, Nischal A, Singh S, Dalal PK. Quality of life and disability in patients with Dhat syndrome: a cross-sectional study. Indian J Psychol Med. 2022;44(5):459–65. https://doi.org/10.1177/02537176221078422.
Sharan P, Hans G. Cultural issues related to ICD-11 mental, behavioural and neurodevelopmental disorders. Consort Psychiatr. 2021;2(2):7–15. https://doi.org/10.17816/CP67.
Sridhar VK, Subramanian K, Menon V. Current nosology of Dhat syndrome and state of evidence. Indian J Health Sex Cult. 2018;4(2):8–14.
Sumathipala A, Siribaddana SH, Bhugra D. Culture-bound syndromes: the story of Dhat syndrome. Br J Psychiatry J Ment Sci. 2004;184:200–9. https://doi.org/10.1192/bjp.184.3.200.
Wig NN. Problems of mental health in India. J Clin Soc Psychiatry. 1960;17:48–53.
Wig NN. An overview of cross-cultural and national issues in psychiatric classification. In: Mezzich JE, Honda Y, Kastrup MC, editors. Psychiatric diagnosis: a world perspective. New York: Springer; 1994. p. 3–10.
World Health Organization. International classification of diseases (ICD-10). Geneva: World Health Organization; 1994.
World Health Organization. International classification of diseases. 11th Revision. 2022. https://icd.who.int/en. Accessed 31 July 2023.

# Chapter 4
# Dhat Syndrome in Indian Traditional Medicine

**Deblina Roy and Shubha Joshi**

## 4.1 Introduction

Dhat syndrome, a psychosomatic condition predominantly observed in South Asian cultures, has garnered significant attention due to its unique cultural underpinnings. This chapter would focus on the traditional aspects of Dhat syndrome, examining its historical origins, cultural context (Malhotra and Wig 1975), and the influence of sociocultural factors on its manifestation and treatment. Comprehensively understanding these traditional underpinnings, valuable insights into the complexities surrounding Dhat syndrome can be gained and it can lead to the development of culturally-sensitive approaches for its management. The Prevalence of "Dhat syndrome" is one of the most common entities among the Culture bound syndromes a recent review of world studies reported that among Culture bound syndromes the prevalence is more than 70% (Strong et al. 2022) in males and among females a similar entity though disputed (non-pathological vaginal discharge); have been reported where is prevalence is around 60% in the rural areas (Tripathi et al. 2021). Dhat syndrome has also been called semen Loss anxiety in much of the literature (Prakash et al. 2018).

D. Roy (✉)
Department of Psychiatry, KGMU, Lucknow, India

S. Joshi
Department of Geriatric Mental Health, KGMU, Lucknow, India

© The Author(s), under exclusive license to Springer Nature Singapore Pte Ltd. 2024

S. K. Kar et al. (eds.), *Dhat Syndrome*,
https://doi.org/10.1007/978-981-99-8870-9_4

## 4.2 Historical Concepts of Dhat Syndrome

To understand Dhat syndrome, it is crucial to delve into its historical origins. Ancient texts and references provide valuable insights into the conceptualization of this condition. For instance, Ayurvedic texts highlight the significance of seminal fluid and its role in overall well-being. Additionally, the cultural influences prevalent during different historical periods have shaped the understanding of Dhat syndrome and influenced its perception among affected individuals. The Ayurvedic concept of Dhat Syndrome is deeply rooted in the South east Asian Sub-continent, across the countries of India, Bangladesh, Pakistan, Afghanistan, Sri Lanka, and Myanmar (Kar and Sarkar 2015).

### *4.2.1 Concepts in Ayurveda*

The Traditional ideologies part of the Ayurvedic system approaches the formation of "dhatus" in the below-mentioned ways.

Dhatus: According to Ayurveda, the body is composed of seven dhatus or tissues, with semen (shukra dhatu) being one of them. Semen is considered a vital fluid that plays a crucial role in overall well-being and vitality (Sharma and Chaudhary 2014).

Ojas: Ojas is the subtle essence of all the bodily tissues, including semen. It represents the vitality and immunity of an individual. The loss of semen is believed to deplete ojas and result in various symptoms associated with Dhat syndrome (Prakash et al. 2014).

Virya: Virya refers to the potency or energy of semen. Ayurveda views semen as a precious substance that should be conserved to maintain optimal health and vitality (Gopal Das et al. 2022).

The formation of semen cascade: Please see Fig. 4.1.

Preservation of semen has been emphasised in various religious texts, first pathological explanation comes from the Charaka Samhita regarding "Shukra Meha" i.e. Passing of semen in the Urine in 1500 BC (Kar and Sarkar 2015). According to the text 'Shukra meha' can be caused by excessive indulgence in masturbation and sexual activities, obstruction in the ejaculation of semen, and sexual intercourse with impassionate (non-consenting) women. Black Magic and overpowering sexual urges can be attributed to Semen loss and its manifestations such as weakness lethargy anxiety etc. (Prakash et al. 2014). It has been emphasised that the condensation of semen from the Rasa (food extracts) to formation of drops of semen (shukra) means loss of nutrients at high levels (Fig. 4.2).

*Shiva Samhita* describes sperms (Virya) as compared with "Seed" falling of seed or sperms can lead to death therefore, emphasis was given to preserving the semen to contain vitality and life force (Jadhav 2004).

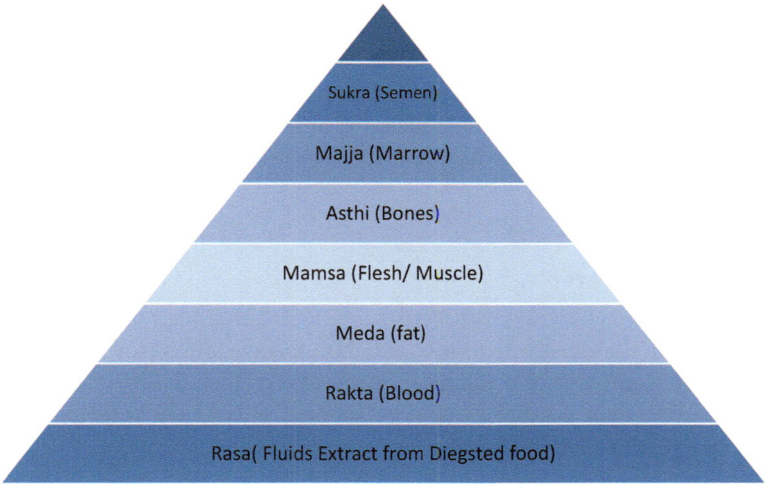


**Fig. 4.1** Formation of semen according to ayurveda and seven essential elements of the Human Body

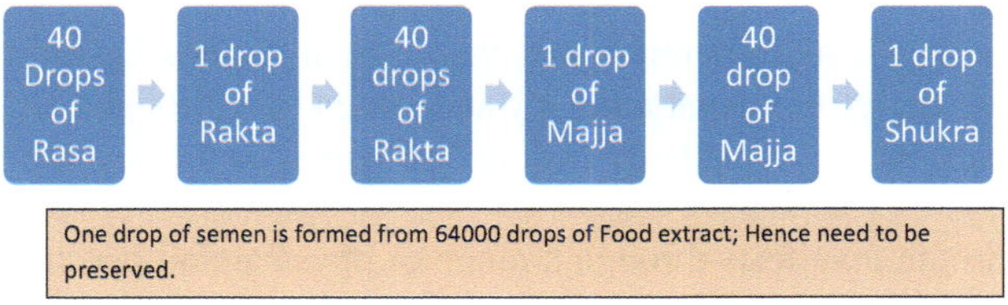


**Fig. 4.2** Formation of semen cascade. Adapted from Sharma and Chaudhary (2014))

## 4.3 Cultural Context of Dhat Syndrome

Culture plays a pivotal role in shaping the beliefs and attitudes surrounding Dhat syndrome. Cultural norms regarding semen and its perceived importance contribute to the development and maintenance of this condition (Strong et al. 2022). Moreover, the conceptualization of masculinity, sexual health, and religious and spiritual beliefs further impact the understanding and experience of Dhat syndrome. As described by various authors culture-bound syndromes such as Dhat Syndrome have different expressions cross-culturally. They have the same phenomenology but have different names across the regions. Therefore the similar phenomenon of Dhat syndrome is called "Prameha" in Srilanka, Shen k'uei in China; Latah in Malaysia; and Imu in Japan (Mehta et al. 2009), and Jiryan in other parts of South East Asia (Simons 1985).

### *4.3.1 Islamic Concept of Dhat Syndrome*

Loss of semen due to masturbation is more harmful than sexual intercourse because the object of arousal is more psychic than that of the actual, which includes sensory modalities of tactile, visual, olfactory and auditory stimulations (Prakash et al. 2014).

### *4.3.2 Buddhist View*

According to the Buddhist way of life sexual intimacy is often frowned upon and is considered a deviation from the spiritual paths (Prakash et al. 2014). therefore loss of semen due to nocturnal emissions is considered an obstacle in the path of spiritual progress (Faure 1998).

### *4.3.3 Christian Philosophies*

Christianity views sexual intercourse as the original sin arising from the story of Adam and Eve, therefore sexual intimacy and semen loss through masturbation and nocturnal emissions are considered sinful contributing to the development of anxiety and guilt.

Dhat syndrome manifests through a range of physical and psychological symptoms. Physical symptoms may include fatigue, weakness, and sexual dysfunction, while psychological symptoms often encompass anxiety, depression, and hypochondriasis. Sociocultural factors, such as cultural stigma and gender roles, can exacerbate the symptomatology of Dhat syndrome and influence its manifestation (Prakash et al. 2014).

## 4.4 Etiology and Causative Factors

### *4.4.1 Traditional Concept*

In traditional concepts, Dhat syndrome is primarily attributed to excessive loss of seminal fluid. It is believed that the loss of vital energy through semen leads to physical and psychological symptoms. Traditional perspectives often associate Dhat syndrome with cultural beliefs, such as the importance of preserving semen for overall well-being and vitality.

### 4.4.2 Modern Concept

Modern concepts of Dhat syndrome consider it a psychosomatic disorder influenced by psychological and social factors. Excessive worry or anxiety about semen loss, cultural and societal beliefs, and underlying psychological conditions like anxiety and depression are considered potential causative factors. Modern understandings focus on the interplay between psychological, cultural, and societal factors in the development and maintenance of Dhat syndrome.

### 4.4.3 Heat Fixation Theory

The concept of food to energy is given importance in Ayurveda therefore it influences the dietary habits in the subcontinent. Certain food items are considered hot and some are considered cold. Traditionally that knowledge is passed down and validated by Ayurvedic practitioners. The food gets sequentially converted into semen/vaginal discharge (Dhatu) through seven stages, and a large quantity of nutritious food is required for the formation of a single drop of semen. It is considered that the 'heat' of the stomach facilitates this conversion of food to semen/vaginal discharge. So, any condition producing heat will hasten this process of conversion, causing excessive semen and vaginal discharge. Therefore the nutrients to nourish the body will get transformed and lost as Semen/Vaginal Discharge leading to weakness, loss of concentration, and several other associated symptoms, hence contributing to overall poor health. This also significantly impacts the reproductive potential of the individual. Therefore according to this concept heat producing food items need to be avoided. Often the person presenting with semen loss (Dhat syndrome) is told about this retrospectively. Treatment is also directed in the form of heating and cooling therapies and abstinence from specific food items as prevention therapies (Joshi et al. 2022). This leads to the avoidance of certain food groups altogether further contributing to ill health (Grover et al. 2016a).

### 4.4.4 The Hollowing/Melting of Bones

This theory again takes reference from the concept of food to dhatus, therefore food to Bone formation uses a lot of precious nutrients from the body. As the individual suffers from semen loss their bones suffer loss hence the symptoms of backache and bone pains, Since the most common attribution is the backbone; backache is commonly reported. This is more common in females additionally due to childbearing and sexual activity there is already weakness, attributing it to semen and vaginal discharge makes it more believable that their bones are hollowing due to semen loss and vaginal discharge.

### 4.4.5 Sex and Masturbation

Historically the age of marriage and initiation of sexual activity was quite young and around the age of puberty. In the old Indian culture premarital sexual activities have been frowned upon, therefore to prevent young people from engaging in such activities it was recommended that abstinence will make them healthier. Whereas the current social structure has changed a lot and the socially acceptable age of sexual initiation has increased with the age restrictions of marriage. Therefore this idea of good health with abstinence does hold to be true anymore. Loss of semen through nocturnal emission, masturbation, urinary loss or any sexual activities happens naturally. But as it is culturally stigmatized it leads to the belief of "loss of sperm causing infertility". The concepts and thoughts surrounding sex and masturbation are the root cause of dhat syndrome. Masturbation is believed to cause an excessive loss of semen, which would then result in a hot body condition and weakness, a condition known in Hindi as *kamjori* (Joshi et al. 2022). Also, masturbation inherently is stigmatized and attributed to later sexual dysfunctions and problems in marital relationships, therefore, complicating the belief systems in the minds of lay people.

The idea of suppressing and avoiding an open discussion of sex and masturbation in society is the foundation of these views. Dhat syndrome is indigenous to that civilizations and nations that are very conservative and support the suppression of sexual impulses. Therefore, it is obvious that the ideas espoused by conservative societies about suppressing and controlling sexual impulses and cravings may be a major factor in the development of Dhat syndrome (Das and Dutt 2020).

### 4.4.6 Stress

In the traditional concept of Dhat syndrome stress is mostly referred to as interpersonal stress and marital conflicts (Roy 2018) and is associated with other physical co-morbidities (Chaturvedi 1988). The stress can be attributed to various reasons which mainly revolve around reproductive and sexual health. Lack of sex and reproductive education complicates it further.

## 4.5 Symptoms and Presentation

The symptoms have been summarised in the following table (Table 4.1). The patients usually attribute the symptoms to semen loss.

**Traditional Concept**: Traditional perspectives of Dhat syndrome primarily focus on physical symptoms associated with the loss of semen, such as fatigue, weakness, and sexual dysfunction. Psychological symptoms, if acknowledged, are

**Table 4.1** Common signs and symptoms of Dhat Syndrome across the sexes

| Physical symptoms | Psychological symptoms | Sexual symptoms |
|---|---|---|
| Backache, body ache, multiple pain symptoms | Low mood | Erectile dysfunction, premature ejaculation |
| Fatigue | Restlessness | Medically unexplained vague symptoms |
| Weakness in bones, eye pain | Lack of concentration | Impotency |
| Indigestion, constipation | Anxiety | Decreased desire, difficulty in arousal and loss of orgasm |
| Listlessness | Forgetfulness | |
| Lack of appetite | Vague psychological symptoms | |

often attributed to physical weakness and imbalance caused by excessive semen loss. The emphasis is more on somatic complaints related to the reproductive system (Chawla 2023; Srinivas 2023).

**Modern Concept**: Modern concepts of Dhat syndrome encompass a broader range of symptoms, including both physical and psychological manifestations. Physical symptoms may include fatigue, weakness, loss of appetite, and sexual dysfunction. Psychological symptoms often encompass anxiety, depression, hypochondriasis, and somatization. Modern perspectives recognize the intricate interplay between the physical and psychological aspects of the syndrome (Dalal et al. 2013; Grover et al. 2016a; Kar and Singh 2017; Tripathi et al. 2021).

## 4.6 Treatment Approaches

### *4.6.1 Traditional Concept*

Traditional treatment approaches for Dhat syndrome mainly revolve around conserving semen and restoring its balance. This involves lifestyle modifications, Ayurvedic therapies, and herbal formulations aimed at rejuvenating the body, strengthening the reproductive system, and addressing underlying imbalances. Traditional perspectives often rely on concepts such as *shukra stambhana* (conservation of semen) and *rasayana* (rejuvenation) therapies.

### *4.6.2 Ayurvedic Treatments for Semen Loss*

Shukra Stambhana (Conservation of Semen): A common treatment method prescribed in Ayurvedic medicine where the loss of semen "Shukra" in both men and women can lead to the development of a lifestyle disease called "*Shukra Kshaya*".

This condition leads to erectile dysfunction, Premature Ejaculation, wrinkling of the skin, muscle pain weakness, multiple somatic symptoms, eye pain, loss of concentration etc. In the "Shukra Stambhana" treatment focus is made on conserving the semen and preventing its loss through any means such as (Masturbation, Night falls, avoiding watching pornography, avoiding multiple partners and engaging in sex only for procreating) this can restore vitality and prevent the above-mentioned symptoms. Conserving semen is often considered to provide sexual vigour and better physical health(Abbot 2023).

"Shukra Stambhana" or semen conservation has also percolated in the current time; often it has become a pop culture event like "no nut November" where people avoid indulging in sexual activities in across a month to preserve semen (Slater 2022).

*Rasayana Therapy*: Rasayana refers to the rejuvenation and revitalization of the body and mind. Specific herbal formulations and dietary recommendations are used to strengthen the reproductive system, restore vitality, and improve overall health (Srinivas 2023).

Rasayana therapy promotes lifespan, enhances mental and intellectual ability, maintains youthfulness, increases lustre, skin glow and body complexion, improves voice health, and maximises the capacity of the body and sense organs. The two primary categories of Rasayana medications are Kamya Rasayana (for enhancing personal health) and Naimittika Rasayana (for treating disorders). The Rasayana medicines, which increase both physical and mental power, include *Amalaki* (Phyllanthus emblica), *Aswagandha* (Withania somnifera), *Brahmi* (Bacopa monnieri), *Shankhapushpi* (Convolvulus pluricaulis), *Guduchi* (Tinospora cordifolia), and *Yastimadhu* (Glycyrrhiza glabra), among others (Srinivas 2023). The treatment also advises abstinence from certain foods like, hot and cold foods thereby reducing certain protein-rich diets to prevent semen loss.

### *4.6.3 Vajikarana Therapy*

Vajikarana aims to enhance sexual potency and reproductive health. It involves the use of aphrodisiac herbs and formulations to strengthen the reproductive system and address any underlying imbalances. This is commonly used in Ashtanga Ayurveda as a treatment for a host of sexual dysfunctions and disorders.

The therapy is preceded by careful adherence to the guidelines outlined in the Ayurvedic texts, numerous body cleaning techniques, and other non-medicinal strategies like conduct, behaviour, and food that promote sexual health. According to Ayurveda, specific tailored herbal and herbo-mineral combinations are given based on a person's nature. Before using these therapies, a number of factors need to be taken into account, including the lack of scientific studies, the potential for adulteration in the herbal and herbo-mineral combinations that are available on the market, and the potential for unforeseen side effects, among others (Dalal et al. 2013).

### *4.6.4 Panchakarma*

Panchakarma is a detoxification and rejuvenation therapy in Ayurveda. It involves various cleansing procedures, such as *basti* (enema) and *virechana* (purgation), to eliminate toxins and restore balance in the body. Panchakarma may be recommended in cases where Dhat syndrome is associated with underlying imbalances or disorders.

Panchkarma therapy involves the following components. *Udarbasti* is commonly used to treat sexual dysfunctions and this aims to restore balance through the following techniques.

Panchkarma Treatment for Erectile Dysfunction

"NASYAM (Applying small drops of medicine through the nose)

VAMANAM (Medicated vomiting)

VIRECHANAM (Medically cleansing the gut through purgation)

BASTI (Medicated enema)

RAKTHAMOKSHAM (Bloodletting) (Chawla 2023)"

This therapy also focuses on semen conservation to be a part of the treatment, also emphasises dietary restrictions and multiple therapies to improve sexual health.

It is important to note that Ayurvedic management of Dhat syndrome should be individualized based on the specific needs and imbalances of the person. Consulting an experienced Ayurvedic practitioner is crucial to receive personalized recommendations and therapies tailored to one's condition.

While Ayurveda offers unique insights into the management of Dhat syndrome, it is essential to integrate Ayurvedic approaches with modern medical interventions and psychotherapy when necessary. A holistic and collaborative approach, combining traditional wisdom with evidence-based practices, can provide comprehensive care for individuals with Dhat syndrome.

### *4.6.5 Modern Concept*

The traditional and modern concepts of Dhat syndrome differ in several ways, including their understanding of the condition's etiology, symptoms, and treatment approaches.

Modern treatment approaches for Dhat syndrome incorporate a multidimensional approach (Prakash et al. 2014; Tripathi et al. 2021). They include psychoeducation, cognitive-behavioural therapy (CBT), medication (if necessary), and supportive counselling (Grover et al. 2016b). The focus is on addressing psychological factors, reducing anxiety and worry related to semen loss, challenging erroneous beliefs, and improving overall mental well-being. Modern interventions often integrate traditional practices with evidence-based approaches for a holistic and comprehensive management plan (Grover et al. 2016b).

## 4.7 Challenges in Treating Dhat Syndrome in Modern Medicine

Treating Dhat syndrome within the modern medical framework poses several challenges. These challenges stem from various factors, including the complex nature of the condition, cultural influences, diagnostic difficulties, and the need for a holistic and culturally sensitive approach. The stigma surrounding sexual health and reluctance to discuss semen-related issues can hinder individuals from seeking help (Farid et al. 2019). Cultural beliefs and misconceptions about the condition may also influence treatment-seeking behaviours and adherence to medical recommendations(Behere and Natraj 1984). The symptoms of Dhat syndrome can overlap with other mental health disorders, such as anxiety, depression, and somatization disorders (Kar and Sarkar 2015). Clinicians need to carefully differentiate between Dhat syndrome and other related conditions to provide appropriate treatment(Trollope-Kumar 2001).

Many healthcare professionals may have limited awareness and training regarding Dhat syndrome, especially outside regions where it is prevalent. This can lead to underrecognition, misinterpretation of symptoms, and inadequate treatment approaches. (Kostick et al. 2010). Integrating these approaches can be challenging, as there may be differences in belief systems, treatment modalities, and cultural contexts. A collaborative approach that respects and incorporates traditional practices while adhering to evidence-based guidelines is crucial (Dalal et al. 2013). Incorporating psychological interventions, such as cognitive-behavioural therapy (CBT), can be vital in addressing anxiety, depression, and cognitive distortions associated with Dhat syndrome(Grover et al. 2016a). Providing holistic care for individuals with Dhat syndrome requires a multidisciplinary approach. Collaboration between psychiatrists, psychologists, primary care physicians, and other healthcare professionals is necessary to address the physical, psychological, and cultural aspects of the condition. However, coordination and collaboration among different healthcare providers can be challenging due to fragmented healthcare systems(Roy 2018).

## 4.8 Conclusion

Addressing these challenges requires a comprehensive and culturally sensitive approach. Increasing awareness, promoting culturally sensitive care, improving diagnostic clarity, enhancing training for healthcare providers, and fostering multidisciplinary collaboration are crucial steps in overcoming the challenges of treating Dhat syndrome within the modern medical framework. Dhat syndrome is a complex condition with cultural influences, diagnostic difficulties, and the need for a holistic and culturally sensitive approach. Clinicians need to differentiate between Dhat syndrome and other mental health disorders to provide appropriate treatment.

Collaboration between psychiatrists, psychologists, primary care physicians, and other healthcare professionals is necessary to address the physical, psychological, and cultural aspects of the condition, but coordination and collaboration among different healthcare providers can be challenging due to fragmented healthcare systems.

## References


Abbot V. Shukra Dhatu: Ayurvedic view of sexual health and fertility [WWW Document]. Lybrate; 2023. https://www.lybrate.com/topic/shukra-dhatu-the-ayurvedic-view-of-sexual-health-and-fertility/ba2df2b911b80405215e56f6b19c8b10. Accessed 13 June 2023.

Behere PB, Natraj GS. Dhat syndrome: the phenomenology of a culture bound sex neurosis of the orient. Indian J Psychiatry. 1984;26:76–8.

Chaturvedi SK. Psychaesthenic syndrome related to leukorrhoea in Indian women. J Psychosom Obstet Gynecol. 1988;8:67–72.

Chawla R. Uttarbasti Panchkarma treatment for erectile dysfunction [WWW Document]. Lybrate; 2023. https://www.lybrate.com/topic/uttarbasti-panchkarma-treatment-for-erectile-dysfunction/139ddae15b3f74e1c28574c5c94696dd. Accessed 13 June 2023.

Dalal PK, Tripathi A, Gupta SK. Vajikarana: treatment of sexual dysfunctions based on Indian concepts. Indian J Psychiatry. 2013;55:S273–6. https://doi.org/10.4103/0019-5545.105550.

Das J, Dutt S. Dhat syndrome and its perceived impact on psychological well-being. Indian J Soc Psychiatr. 2020;36:136. https://doi.org/10.4103/ijsp.ijsp_22_19.

Farid M, Barandouzi ZA, Valipour NS. Knowledge, attitudes, and coping strategies regarding pubertal changes among adolescent girls: risks and compliances for health promotion in puberty. J Educ Health Promot. 2019;8:176. https://doi.org/10.4103/jehp.jehp_381_18.

Faure B. The red thread: Buddhist approaches to sexuality. Princeton University Press; 1998.

Gopal Das C, Ananta Kalyan D, Rao AB, Jog A. Management approaches to Dhat syndrome: a review. IJHSC. 2022;8:55–64. https://doi.org/10.5281/zenodo.6806037.

Grover S, Avasthi A, Gupta S, Dan A, Tripathi A, Chakravatri K, Rao TS. Phenomenology and beliefs of patients with Dhat syndrome: a nationwide multicentric study. Indian J Soc Psychiatry. 2016a;62:57–66. https://doi.org/10.1177/0020764015591857.

Grover S, Gupta S, Mahajan S, Avasthi A. Pathway of care among patients with Dhat syndrome attending a psychosexual clinic in tertiary care center in North India. Ind Psychiatry J. 2016b;25:72.

Jadhav S. Dhāt syndrome: a re-evaluation. Psychiatry. 2004;3:14–6. https://doi.org/10.1383/psyt.3.8.14.43399. Unusual Psychiatric Syndromes.

Joshi S, Tripathi A, Agarwal S, Singh N, Gupta B, Nischal A, Kar SK. Phenomenology, disability and sexual functioning in female Dhat syndrome: a study of tertiary care gynaecology outpatients. Gen Psychiatr. 2022;35:e100863. https://doi.org/10.1136/gpsych-2022-100863.

Kar SK, Sarkar S. Dhat syndrome: evolution of concept, current understanding, and need of an integrated approach. J Hum Reprod Sci. 2015;8:130–4. https://doi.org/10.4103/0974-1208.165143.

Kar SK, Singh A. Where lies the fault in diagnosing dhat syndrome among females? Understanding through a case study. Indian J Psychol Med. 2017;39:506–8.

Kostick KM, Schensul SL, Jadhav K, Singh R, Bavadekar A, Saggurti N. Treatment seeking, vaginal discharge and psychosocial distress among women in urban Mumbai. Cult Med Psychiatry. 2010;34:529–47.

Malhotra HK, Wig NN. Dhat syndrome: a culture-bound sex neurosis of the orient. Arch Sex Behav. 1975;4:519–28.

Mehta V, De A, Balachandran C. Dhat syndrome: a reappraisal. Indian J Dermatol. 2009;54:89–90. https://doi.org/10.4103/0019-5154.49002.

Prakash O, Kar SK, Sathyanarayana Rao TS. Indian story on semen loss and related Dhat syndrome. Indian J Psychiatry. 2014;56:377–82. https://doi.org/10.4103/0019-5545.146532.
Prakash S, Sharan P, Sood M. A qualitative study on psychopathology of dhat syndrome in men: implications for classification of disorders. Asian J Psychiatr. 2018;35:79–88.
Roy D. Female Dhat syndrome: a condition beyond just vaginal discharge. IJHSC. 2018;4:16–22.
Sharma V, Chaudhary AK. Concepts of Dhatu Siddhanta (theory of tissues formation and differentiation) and Rasayana; probable predecessor of stem cell therapy. Ayu. 2014;35:231. https://doi.org/10.4103/0974-8520.153731.
Simons RC. Sorting the culture-bound syndromes. In: Simons RC, Hughes CC, editors. The culture-bound syndromes: folk illnesses of psychiatric and anthropological interest, culture, illness, and healing. Dordrecht: Springer; 1985. p. 25–38. https://doi.org/10.1007/978-94-009-5251-5_2.
Slater J. What is No Nut November and what are the rules? | Metro News [WWW Document]. Metro News; 2022. https://metro.co.uk/2022/10/31/what-is-no-nut-november-and-what-are-the-rules-17662259/. Accessed 13 June 2023.
Srinivas P. Rasayana (Ayurvedic Rejuvenation Therapy) | CCRAS | Ministry of AYUSH (Govt. of India) [WWW Document]. Central Council for Research in Ayurvedic Sciences; 2023. http://ccras.nic.in/content/rasayana-ayurvedic-rejuvenation-therapy. Accessed 13 June 2023.
Strong YN, Li A, White ME, Razzak AN, Anderson DJ, Kaye AD, Herron EW, Khater NP, Cornett EM, Urits I. Dhat syndrome: epidemiology, risk factors, comorbidities, diagnosis, treatment, and management. Health Psychol Res. 2022;10:38759. https://doi.org/10.52965/001c.38759.
Tripathi A, Roy D, Kar SK. Distress due to nonpathological vaginal discharge: a new face of Dhat syndrome in females. J Psychosex Health. 2021;3:315–21. https://doi.org/10.1177/26318318211049547.
Trollope-Kumar K. Cultural and biomedical meanings of the complaint of leukorrhea in South Asian women. Tropical Med Int Health. 2001;6:260–6.

# Chapter 5
# Course and Outcome of Dhat Syndrome

**Surendra Singh Rajpurohit and Naresh Nebhinani**

## 5.1 Introduction

Dhat syndrome (DS), a psychosomatic condition commonly seen in the Indian subcontinent, is characterized by preoccupation with loss of vital fluid (Dhat), due to which a person believes that it is resulting in various physical and psychological symptoms in them. Individuals experiencing Dhat syndrome attribute their physical and mental distress and, at times, comorbid depressive and anxiety symptoms to the perceived loss of semen through nocturnal emissions, urination, or other means. Professor N. N. Wig is credited with coining "Dhat syndrome" in 1960. (Rao 2021) However, in different cultural contexts, similar symptoms or beliefs are referred to by other names, like "Jiryan" in South East Asia, "Prameha" in Sri Lanka, and "Shen k'uei" in China, reflecting the cultural and linguistic diversity in different regions where similar conditions are observed. (Kar and Sarkar 2015; Mehta et al. 2009).

In the *International Classification of Diseases (ICD-10)*, Dhat syndrome was categorized as both a neurotic disorder (code F48.8) and a culture-specific disorder (Annex 2) resulting from "undue concern about the debilitating effects of the passage of semen" (World Health Organization 2004). In the glossary section of DSM-5 it is categorized as a "cultural concept of distress" (American Psychiatric Association 2013).

S. S. Rajpurohit · N. Nebhinani (✉)
Department of Psychiatry, AIIMS Jodhpur, Jodhpur, India

© The Author(s), under exclusive license to Springer Nature Singapore Pte Ltd. 2024
S. K. Kar et al. (eds.), *Dhat Syndrome*,
https://doi.org/10.1007/978-981-99-8870-9_5

## 5.2 Age of Onset

Regarding the prevalence rate of Dhat syndrome, as per a systematic review by Udina et al., it is estimated that around 7% of patients seen in sexual health clinics in India have Dhat syndrome (Udina et al. 2013). In a study done in Karnataka, India, the prevalence rate was around 12.5% (Rao et al. 1997).

Generally, it is seen that the onset of Dhat syndrome occurs in young adulthood. In different studies, the mean age of onset of Dhat syndrome varies from 18 to 30 years (Grover et al. 2015; Rao et al. 1997; Shahi et al. 2022). In female patients diagnosed with Dhat syndrome, studies have found that the average age of onset tends to be higher than males, typically between 23 and 36 years (Joshi et al. 2022; Mehra et al. 2021; Strong et al. 2022). In a systematic review of 11 studies including 805 patients with Dhat syndrome, the mean age of patients was 26 years (Udina et al. 2013). In males with Dhat syndrome, it has been observed that individuals with comorbid sexual and other psychiatric conditions tend to have a later onset than those without any comorbidities (Shahi et al. 2022). On the contrary, Shahi et al. found no correlation between the duration of symptoms and the presence or absence of comorbidity in patients with Dhat syndrome (Shahi et al. 2022).

## 5.3 Risk Factors

Various studies have tried to identify different risk factors associated with Dhat syndrome. Ranjith and Mohan (2006) proposed an integrated model that considers psychological and sociocultural factors in understanding Dhat syndrome. It tries to provide a comprehensive framework for understanding the condition by considering both individual psychological factors and the influence of sociocultural factors on its development and manifestation (Ranjith and Mohan 2006).

Lower or middle socioeconomic status is often identified as a risk factor for developing Dhat syndrome (Bagadia et al. 1972; Behere and Natraj 1984; Bhatia and Malik 1991; Deb and Balhara 2013). According to a study by Malhotra and Wig, compared to people from lower social classes, individuals from higher social classes tend to engage more openly in discussions about sex. They are also less fearful regarding any possible health-related adverse effects which may result due to semen loss. Whereas people from lower social classes tend to view sex as a taboo subject, they do not discuss it. These factors lead to a lack of information about normal sexual processes, which can cause the person to believe that nocturnal emissions are abnormal (Malhotra and Wig 1975).

Different studies show that among patients with Dhat syndrome, generally, a conservative attitude towards sex is present (Bhatia and Malik 1991; Strong et al. 2022). Furthermore, individuals who are unmarried or recently married and reside in rural areas are more commonly affected by Dhat syndrome (Strong et al. 2022). A survey conducted in Patiala (a district in northern India) found that many people from rural backgrounds and college graduates perceived that excessive sexual activity and masturbation are detrimental and can potentially result in mental illness (Singh 1985). This lack of appropriate sexual education is a significant risk factor for the development of Dhat syndrome among such people. Certain studies suggest that a person's educational status does not influence if they develop Dhat syndrome (Kendurkar et al. 2008).

The individual's cultural beliefs have been observed to influence the development of Dhat syndrome significantly. These cultural interpretations attribute the underlying pathology of Dhat syndrome to various prevailing sociocultural teachings. In some cultural groups, the loss of semen is interpreted as a representation of illness, misfortune, or maladaptive behaviour (MacFarland et al. 2017). As per Ayurveda, of the seven elements (Dhatu) in the human body, semen is the most refined one (Obeyesekere 1977). Ancient texts emphasizing the importance of abstinence also suggest that forty meals result in a drop of blood, forty drops of blood lead to one drop of bone marrow, and forty drops of marrow culminate in one drop of semen (Bhugra 1992; Malhotra and Wig 1975). As a result of such sociocultural beliefs, the loss of semen is perceived as a significant concern that causes distress in the individual, thereby impacting their libido and sexual functions. This type of cultural understanding by the patient also leads the patient to think that fatigue and any other physical symptoms he/she experiences are due to the loss of semen from their body (Ranjith and Mohan 2006). Nevertheless, industrialization and urbanization have recently resulted in a decline in the stigma surrounding semen loss. Additionally, more accessible factual information about sex, masturbation, and semen loss has decreased the negative psychological responses associated with the loss of semen (MacFarland et al. 2017).

Generally, friends, relatives, colleagues, roadside advertisements, and magazines are familiar sources from which patients obtain information regarding the loss of semen and its associated consequences (Prakash et al. 2018). Several studies have explored DS patients' beliefs towards the factors responsible for their condition. Behere and Natraj conducted interviews with 50 DS patients, in which 52% attributed the cause to masturbation, 16% to engaging in sexual relations before marriage, and 14% to engage in sexual relations outside of marriage (Behere and Natraj 1984). Similarly, in a multicentric study involving 780 patients across India, many of the patients believed that loss of semen was due to excessive masturbation (55%) by them. They also ascribed it to factors such as sexual dreams, excessive sexual desire, consumption of high-energy foods, and past wrong-doings during early childhood, among other reasons (Grover et al. 2016a). Female DS patients believed they had vaginal discharge because they consumed warm foods and drinks or an imbalanced diet. Other reasons stated by female DS patients included stress, various emotional factors, infections, and excessive heat in their bodies due to warm weather (Mehra et al. 2021).

Based on all the risk factors, an etiological model is constructed to illustrate how various factors predispose an individual to the development of Dhat syndrome, as depicted in Fig. 5.1. Upon entering puberty, nocturnal emissions and masturbatory

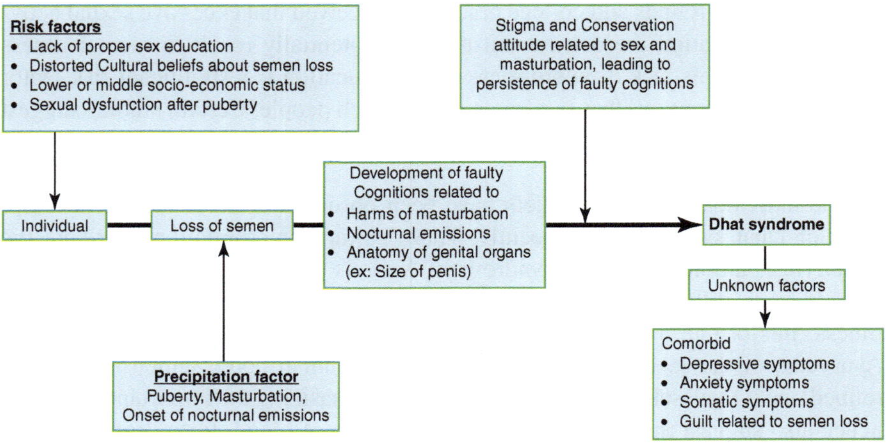


**Fig. 5.1** Etiological model of Dhat syndrome

practices result in the perceived loss of semen in an individual. This perception, combined with the influence of various risk factors and cultural beliefs regarding the detrimental effects of semen loss, leads to distorted cognitions in the individual. Moreover, societal stigma and the individual's conservative attitudes toward sexual activities hinder acquiring the accurate knowledge necessary to correct these distorted beliefs—consequently, the individual experiences significant distress, culminating in the manifestation of Dhat syndrome.

## 5.4 Comorbidities

In the context of Dhat syndrome, comorbidity commonly refers to the coexistence of Dhat syndrome with other psychiatric or sexual disorders. Several studies have explored the relationship between Dhat syndrome and different psychiatric disorders and sexual dysfunctions. Depression, sexual dysfunction like premature ejaculation, and erectile dysfunction are common in patients with Dhat syndrome.

As per review articles, depression and anxiety are the most commonly reported comorbidities. The prevalence rate of depression and anxiety has been seen to range from 40 to 66% and 21 to 38%, respectively, among different studies. Somatoform and hypochondriacal disorders are reported to be in the range of 32–40% (Deb and Balhara 2013; Udina et al. 2013). Approximately 50% of individuals with Dhat syndrome experience sexual dysfunction in the form of premature ejaculation and erectile dysfunction (Grover et al. 2015; Udina et al. 2013). Other less frequently observed comorbidities in individuals with Dhat syndrome include phobias, stress reactions, obsessive-compulsive disorders, body dysmorphic disorders, and delusional disorders (Deb and Balhara 2013; Kar et al. 2017).

A retrospective study including 264 DS patients from a psychosexual clinic in a tertiary care centre had seen that 27.3% of patients had some psychiatric comorbidity. Among them, 15.1% of patients had depressive disorder, and 12.9% had anxiety, neurotic, and stress-related disorder as per ICD 10. One-third of the patients had comorbid sexual dysfunction, premature ejaculation in 22.7% and erectile dysfunction in 20.4% as per ICD 10 (Grover et al. 2015).

Grover et al. assessed 780 DS patients across 15 centres in India about the main consequences they were experiencing due to the passage of Dhat. Most of them (75.6%) reported experiencing weakness in their sexual ability because of loss of vitality in the form of semen. Other expected consequences included loss of beauty, reduction in penile size, and risk of dying early (Grover et al. 2016a).

In a study conducted on female patients with Dhat syndrome, using the *Hospital Anxiety and Depression Rating Scale (HADS*), abnormal levels of depression were found in 18.6% of patients. In comparison, anxiety disorder was observed in 10% of patients. Additionally, based on the DSM-5 criteria, 7.1% of Dhat syndrome patients were diagnosed with Somatic Symptom Disorder (Joshi et al. 2022). In a special clinic-based study, about 7% of DS patients reported having comorbid substance use disorders, which is similar to rates of substance use disorder seen in any other urban general medical setting or other population groups (Olfson et al. 2000; Prakash et al. 2016).

The high rate of depressive and anxiety disorder in DS patients has been attributed to the significant guilt experienced by the patient due to the loss of semen. It can be attributed to the socio-cultural beliefs of the patients, where the loss of semen is perceived as the loss of the "vital elixir of life." According to this belief, the loss of semen can deplete the body of its energy, resulting in physical consequences such as impotence, infertility, and mental weakness (Singh 1985).

## 5.5 Duration of Illness and Pathway of Care

It is seen that patients with DS generally take a long time to initiate treatment seeking from any health care professionals. When individuals with Dhat syndrome initially seek help for their condition, they predominantly choose primarily indigenous healers as their first point of contact. They may also turn to friends or relatives, traditional faith healers, allopathic doctors, and sometimes pharmacists for assistance (Singh et al. 2016). Among indigenous practitioners, Ayurvedic doctors are the most preferred choice. Patients may take up to 6–7 years before consulting any health care professional, during which, on average, they seek 2–3 consultations from indigenous practitioners (Grover et al. 2016c; Singh et al. 2016). The only factor observed to be linked to earlier consultation from a healthcare professional for treatment is the absence of any comorbid sexual dysfunction (Grover et al. 2016c).

It is suggested that the most prevalent obstacles in seeking help from mental health professionals are lack of knowledge, awareness of psychosexual disorders, limited accessibility to psychiatric services, and stigma related to the condition (Singh et al. 2016). Additionally, beliefs such as the absence of available cures or the perception that the symptoms are not severe enough hinder the individuals from seeking assistance. Misinformation provided by indigenous practitioners may also be one reason for delayed presentation to specialized Psychosexual clinics (Grover et al. 2016c).

Similarly, a significant delay in consultation is reported in female patients with DS. (Joshi et al. 2022). It might be due to the limited availability of qualified healthcare professionals in rural areas. However, in contrast, most patients (72.9%) believe that the disease could be relieved through treatment by a medical practitioner.

A Community-level study of 1777 individuals with Dhat syndrome reported that around 73% of patients consulted hakims (50%) and homeopaths. Only one-fourth of the patient sought treatment from either physician (18.6%), psychiatrist (1.6%), psychologist (0.7%), urologist (0.3%), or infertility specialist (5.6%) (Khan 2005).

When patients consult with non-allopathic practitioners, it can reinforce misconceptions surrounding semen loss, amplifying their fear and anxiety. This, in turn, prompts them to seek assistance from multiple care providers, resulting in repeated visits and significant investments of time, effort, and money, all without experiencing significant symptom relief. This situation highlights the substantial amount of time lost in the pursuit of appropriate healthcare. The constant cycle of seeking advice, experiencing heightened fear and anxiety, and consulting various care providers leads patients to invest significant resources without finding relief for their symptoms (Singh et al. 2016).

Several studies have explored the mean duration of illness, time to help-seeking from medical professionals, and their association with pathways of care (Grover et al. 2016c; Khan 2005) In males with Dhat syndrome, the duration of illness has been around 5 years (Grover et al. 2016c; Shahi et al. 2022; Singh et al. 2016) and around 6 years in females.(Joshi et al. 2022; Mehra et al. 2021).

## 5.6 Dropout Rates

The definition of dropout rate varies across different studies examining Dhat syndrome. In some studies, the dropout rate is defined as non-completion of the predetermined treatment or if a patient discontinues treatment before the specified follow-up duration intended for assessment. Additionally, a few studies consider a patient as having dropped out if they fail to attend any further follow-up visits after the initial one (Bhatia and Malik 1991; Grover et al. 2016b; Singh 1985).

One of the primary reasons for the high dropout rate in Dhat syndrome treatment has been attributed to patients' dissatisfaction with the explanations given regarding their illness and the statement that semen loss is not truly harmful. Another possibility suggested is that some patients may experience rapid recovery, leading them to forego follow-up appointments (Chadda and Ahuja 1990).

A significant dropout rate, reaching as high as 60%, has been observed among individuals with Dhat syndrome who seek treatment (Grover et al. 2016b; Singh 1985). Additionally, some studies have suggested a higher dropout rate among patients receiving counselling alone than those receiving some form of medication (Bhatia and Malik 1991). Patients often switch not only between different doctors but also between different systems of medicine. Many patients consider indigenous medicines, advice of hakims, and herbal remedies a better treatment modality for Dhat syndrome. Additionally, some patients believe that dietary interventions such as consuming ghee (butter), protein and iron-rich foods, milk, receiving vitamin injections, getting married, hormonal injections, and using aphrodisiacs may be potential remedies (Deb and Balhara 2013).

In a 6-month follow-up study by Grover et al., only 36% of DS patients completed their treatment (Grover et al. 2016b). Early dropout patients (who had dropped out after just one treatment visit) reported the most common reason for treatment discontinuation (42.8%) as the inability to find time for consultations and a lack of prescribed medications from their treating physicians. Other reasons included their perception that it was not a psychiatric issue and their lack of desire for treatment from a psychiatrist. Among patients who sought multiple consultations but did not complete the pre-determined treatment, the most frequently mentioned reason was the lack of improvement in their symptoms (40.7%) (Grover et al. 2016b). It was seen that the source of referral for treatment was the only variable associated with retention in treatment, i.e., patients who are referred from other medical professionals to a psychiatrist are more at risk for dropping out of treatment. And patients who visit psychiatrists directly by themselves are more likely to complete their treatment. It has been seen that treatment completion doesn't depend on any of the socio-demographic variables of patients with DS.

A strong desire of patients with DS for medications was also seen in another study in which 93.5% of patients reported willingness for some medication to treat their illness (Bhatia and Malik 1991). In such cases, it is suggested that therapists should inquire about the patient's expectations of the treatment. It is also recommended that patients who express a strong desire for medication, in addition to ongoing treatment or therapy, should be provided with a prescription (such as a placebo-like multivitamin). This approach may validate the patient's belief in a medical approach to address their symptoms. It is also crucial for psychiatrists who attend to patients with Dhat syndrome, especially those referred by other specialists, to allocate sufficient time to educate patients about the current understanding of Dhat syndrome and the various treatment approaches involved (Grover et al. 2016b).

## 5.7 Treatment of Dhat Syndrome

Existing literature on managing Dhat syndrome mainly consists of case reports and cross-sectional studies, highlighting a research gap for definitive guidelines and treatment algorithms (Deb and Balhara 2013; Raj et al. 1998; Salam et al. 2012). Studies have shown positive treatment outcomes with medications such as lorazepam and imipramine, psychoeducation, and minor tranquillizers (Behere and Natraj 1984; Bhatia and Malik 1991). Comorbid depression in Dhat syndrome patients responded well to fluoxetine (Dhikav et al. 2008). Psychoeducation and culturally informed cognitive-behavioural therapy have been recommended as effective modalities. Treatment approaches also include relaxation therapy, sex education, and a comprehensive approach involving cognitive-behavioural therapy (Avasthi et al. 2017; Chadda and Ahuja 1990; Deb and Balhara 2013). Patient education, correcting cognitive distortions, and addressing psychological and physiological aspects of Dhat syndrome are crucial for symptom improvement. Innovative interventions, such as using models and diagrams for patient education and challenging beliefs, have shown promising results (Chavan et al. 2009). Cognitive-behavioural therapy consisting of multiple sessions focusing on education, cognitive restructuring, relaxation exercises, and homework assignments has been effective. These interventions emphasize the importance of addressing patient beliefs, providing education, and addressing both psychological and physiological factors to promote symptom remission and overall well-being (Innamuri and Ramaswamy 2021; Salam et al. 2012).

As highlighted in various studies, convincing patients about the psychological origins of Dhat syndrome, which are culturally unfamiliar to them, is often considered the most significant challenge in its treatment. Overcoming this hurdle requires a gradual approach, and there is a need for innovative and novel approaches to address it more effectively in the future (Prakash and Mandal 2014).

## 5.8 Prognosis

The diagnostic stability of Dhat syndrome has been a subject of debate and scrutiny. While some studies suggest that the syndrome shows stability over time, others indicate significant diagnostic variability. The lack of consensus on specific diagnostic criteria and the cultural variations in symptom presentation contribute to this diagnostic uncertainty (Deb and Balhara 2013).

A study was conducted to assess the diagnostic stability and naturalistic longitudinal outcome of 36 patients with Dhat syndrome diagnosed according to the DSM-IV criteria (Sameer 2015). They were interviewed after 6–10 years of their Initial medical consultation. It was seen that 63% of patients didn't meet the Dhat syndrome criteria any longer. Still, most of these patients instead met the criteria for either somatoform disorder (47%), generalised anxiety disorder (17%), or depressive disorder (8%). Only 26% of DS patients had achieved clinical remission. It was also observed that individuals who no longer fulfil the diagnostic criteria for Dhat syndrome are significantly more likely to be married and older than those who continue to experience Dhat syndrome later in their lives (Sameer 2015).

At the community level, Khan (2005) found that out of the 1777 DS patients visiting different health professionals, 60% reported being concerned about the loss of semen for only 6 months (Khan 2005). It was also seen that only 14% of patients had DS for more than 2 years, which may indicate the possibility of early remission of symptoms in the community population (Khan 2005).

Contrasting findings have also been reported regarding the persistence of symptoms for a longer duration. For instance, De Silva and Dissanayake found that the duration of symptoms related to semen loss experienced by patients with DS in their study ranged from 6 months to 20 years, with a mean duration of about 5 years (De Silva and Dissanayake 1989). Generally, it is observed that patients are likely to experience Dhat syndrome for a duration ranging from 4.5 to 6.25 years (Grover et al. 2016c; Joshi et al. 2022; Mehra et al. 2021; Shahi et al. 2022).

A varying treatment response rate has been noted in most studies where any form of intervention is employed. Behere and Natraj observed that out of 50 DS patients who received the intervention (psychoeducation, minor tranquillizers), approximately two-thirds completely recovered over 1 year. (Behere and Natraj 1984) On the other hand, Grover et al. found that after 6 months of treatment using pharmacological and non-pharmacological methods, only 21% of patients achieved complete recovery. More than 40% of the patients did not perceive any change in their symptoms (Grover et al. 2016b). It highlights the importance of conducting comprehensive research and developing novel and enhanced treatment strategies that may demonstrate greater effectiveness in managing the condition.

A case study has suggested that excessive distress associated with worry over semen loss in DS patients may even contribute to the development of more severe psychiatric conditions such as schizophrenia. It has been proposed that the stress from semen loss while disrupting the hypothalamic-pituitary-adrenal axis may cause epigenetic changes. This may result in the transformation of a prodromal phase to schizophrenia (Kar et al. 2017).

Compared to healthy people, a lower quality of life (QoL) is seen in patients with Dhat syndrome. In a study comparing 117 DS patients with matched control, poor QoL was seen in all the domains (physical, psychological, environmental, and social health) of the WHO QOL-BREF scale. It is also seen that DS patients with psychiatric or sexual comorbid conditions have a poorer QoL compared to those without any comorbidities. It could be attributed to the considerable psychological distress caused by their symptoms, impairing their daily functioning. Similarly, a significantly higher rate of disability as per the World Health Organization Disability Assessment Schedule (WHODAS) is also seen in patients with DS compared to healthy controls, with DS patients with comorbid conditions having even more, higher levels of disability than those without comorbidities (Shahi et al. 2022).

## 5.9 Conclusions

Dhat syndrome is a psychosomatic condition commonly observed in the Indian subcontinent. Lower or middle socioeconomic status, conservative attitudes towards sex, and being unmarried are identified risk factors associated with DS. Cultural beliefs held by individuals coupled with the impact of various risk factors results in the development of distorted cognitions related to semen loss in the patient and eventual development of DS. Common comorbidities reported in individuals with DS include depression, anxiety, and sexual dysfunction. Patients may delay seeking professional help for an average duration of 6–7 years, during which they typically consult with indigenous practitioners. Psychoeducation and culturally informed cognitive-behavioural therapy form the mainstay of treatment approaches for DS. However, the high dropout rate poses a significant challenge in the treatment of DS. Regarding the long-term course of the condition, there is considerable diagnostic variability. Moreover, there is a possibility of early remission of symptoms within the community population.

## References

American Psychiatric Association, editor. Diagnostic and statistical manual of mental disorders: DSM-5. 5th ed. American Psychiatric Association; 2013.

Avasthi A, Grover S, Sathyanarayana Rao TS. Clinical practice guidelines for management of sexual dysfunction. Indian J Psychiatry. 2017;59(Suppl 1):S91–S115. https://doi.org/10.4103/0019-5545.196977.

Bagadia V, Dave K, Pradhan P, Shah L. A study of 258 male patients with sexual problems/1. Indian J Psychiatry. 1972;14(2):143–51.

Behere PB, Natraj GS. Dhat syndrome: the phenomenology of a culture bound sex neurosis of the orient. Indian J Psychiatry. 1984;26(1):76–8.

Bhatia MS, Malik SC. Dhat syndrome—a useful diagnostic entity in Indian culture. Br J Psychiatry J Ment Sci. 1991;159:691–5. https://doi.org/10.1192/bjp.159.5.691.

Bhugra D. Psychiatry in ancient Indian texts: a review. Hist Psychiatry. 1992;3(10):167–86. https://doi.org/10.1177/0957154X9200301002.

Chadda RK, Ahuja N. Dhat syndrome. A sex neurosis of the Indian subcontinent. Br J Psychiatry J Ment Sci. 1990;156:577–9. https://doi.org/10.1192/bjp.156.4.577.

Chavan B, Kaur J, Singla M, Sharma A. Non-pharmacological treatment of Dhat syndrome. J Ment Health Hum Behav. 2009;14(2):69–73.

Deb KS, Balhara YPS. Dhat syndrome: a review of the world literature. Indian J Psychol Med. 2013;35(4):326–31. https://doi.org/10.4103/0253-7176.122219.

De Silva P, Dissanayake SAW. The use of semen syndrome in Sri Lanka: A clinical study. Sex Marital Ther. 1989;4:195–204.

Dhikav V, Aggarwal N, Gupta S, Jadhavi R, Singh K. Depression in Dhat syndrome. J Sex Med. 2008;5(4):841–4. https://doi.org/10.1111/j.1743-6109.2007.00481.x.

Grover S, Gupta S, Mehra A, Avasthi A. Comorbidity, knowledge and attitude towards sex among patients with Dhat syndrome: a retrospective study. Asian J Psychiatr. 2015;17:50–5. https://doi.org/10.1016/j.ajp.2015.07.002.

Grover S, Avasthi A, Gupta S, Dan A, Neogi R, Behere PB, Lakdawala B, Tripathi A, Chakraborty K, Sinha V, Bhatia MS, Patjoshi A, Rao TSS, Rozatkar A. Phenomenology and beliefs of patients with Dhat syndrome: a nationwide multicentric study. Int J Soc Psychiatry. 2016a;62(1):57–66. https://doi.org/10.1177/0020764015591857.

Grover S, Gupta S, Avasthi A. A follow-up study of patients with Dhat syndrome: treatment pattern, outcome, and reasons for dropout from treatment. Indian J Psychiatry. 2016b;58(1):49–56. https://doi.org/10.4103/0019-5545.174373.

Grover S, Gupta S, Mahajan S, Avasthi A. Pathway of care among patients with Dhat syndrome attending a psychosexual clinic in tertiary care center in North India. Ind Psychiatry J. 2016c;25(1):72–7. https://doi.org/10.4103/0972-6748.196040.

Innamuri R, Ramaswamy D. Demystifying Dhat syndrome: a two-session therapy proposal. J Psychosexual Health. 2021;3(3):270–4.

Joshi S, Tripathi A, Agarwal S, Singh N, Gupta B, Nischal A, Kar SK. Phenomenology, disability and sexual functioning in female Dhat syndrome: a study of tertiary care gynaecology outpatients. Gen Psychiatr. 2022;35(5):e100863. https://doi.org/10.1136/gpsych-2022-100863.

Kar S, Sarkar S. Dhat syndrome: evolution of concept, current understanding, and need of an integrated approach. J Hum Reprod Sci. 2015;8(3):130. https://doi.org/10.4103/0974-1208.165143.

Kar SK, Shahi MK, Tripathi A. Dhat syndrome as the prodrome of schizophrenia: understanding the cultural distress. Asian J Psychiatr. 2017;25:203–4. https://doi.org/10.1016/j.ajp.2016.11.006.

Kendurkar A, Kaur B, Agarwal AK, Singh H, Agarwal V. Profile of adult patients attending a marriage and sex clinic in India. Int J Soc Psychiatry. 2008;54(6):486–93. https://doi.org/10.1177/0020764008090795.

Khan N. Dhat syndrome in relation to demographic characteristics. Indian J Psychiatry. 2005;47(1):54. https://doi.org/10.4103/0019-5545.46077.

MacFarland AS, Al-Maashani M, Al Busaidi Q, Al-Naamani A, El-Bouri M, Al-Adawi S. Culture-specific pathogenicity of Dhat (semen loss) syndrome in an Arab/Islamic Society, Oman. Oman Med J. 2017;32(3):251–5. https://doi.org/10.5001/omj.2017.47.

Malhotra HK, Wig NN. Dhat syndrome: a culture-bound sex neurosis of the orient. Arch Sex Behav. 1975;4(5):519–28. https://doi.org/10.1007/BF01542130.

Mehra A, Kathirvel S, Gainder S, Avasthi A, Grover S. Female Dhat syndrome in primary care setting. Ind Psychiatry J. 2021;30(2):278–84. https://doi.org/10.4103/ipj.ipj_76_20.

Mehta V, De A, Balachandran C. Dhat syndrome: a reappraisal. Indian J Dermatol. 2009;54(1):89. https://doi.org/10.4103/0019-5154.49002.

Obeyesekere G. The theory and practice of psychological medicine in the Ayurvedic tradition. Cult Med Psychiatry. 1977;1(2):155–81. https://doi.org/10.1007/BF00114848.

Olfson M, Shea S, Feder A, Fuentes M, Nomura Y, Gameroff M, Weissman MM. Prevalence of anxiety, depression, and substance use disorders in an urban general medicine practice. Arch Fam Med. 2000;9(9):876–83. https://doi.org/10.1001/archfami.9.9.876.

Prakash S, Mandal P. Culture-bound syndromes: nosological and management issues. Indian J Psychiatry. 2014;56(1):99. https://doi.org/10.4103/0019-5545.124739.

Prakash S, Sharan P, Sood M. A study on phenomenology of Dhat syndrome in men in a general medical setting. Indian J Psychiatry. 2016;58(2):129–41. https://doi.org/10.4103/0019-5545.183776.

Prakash S, Sharan P, Sood M. A qualitative study on psychopathology of dhat syndrome in men: Implications for classification of disorders. Asian J Psychiatr. 2018;35:79–88. https://doi.org/10.1016/j.ajp.2018.05.007. Epub 2018 May 18. PMID: 29803962.

Raj A, Prasadarao P, Raguram R. Cognitive behaviour therapy in Dhat syndrome: a case study. Indian J Clin Psychol. 1998;25(2):211–7.

Ranjith G, Mohan R. Dhat syndrome as a functional somatic syndrome: developing a sociosomatic model. Psychiatry. 2006;69(2):142–50. https://doi.org/10.1521/psyc.2006.69.2.142.

Rao TSS. History and mystery of Dhat syndrome: a critical look at the current understanding and future directions. Indian J Psychiatry. 2021;63(4):317–25. https://doi.org/10.4103/psychiatry.IndianJPsychiatry_791_20.

Rao T, Rao V, Arif M, Rajendra P, Murthy K, Gangadhar T. Sexual problems in medical practice: a study on its prevalence in an out patient setting. Indian J Psychiatry. 1997;39:53–198.

Salam KPA, Sharma MP, Prakash O. Development of cognitive-behavioral therapy intervention for patients with Dhat syndrome. Indian J Psychiatry. 2012;54(4):367–74. https://doi.org/10.4103/0019-5545.104826.

Sameer M. Is 'pure' Dhat syndrome a stable diagnostic entity? A naturalistic long term follow up study from a tertiary care centre. J Clin Diagn Res. 2015;9(8):VC01–3. https://doi.org/10.7860/JCDR/2015/13399.6275.

Shahi MK, Tripathi A, Singh A, Kar SK, Nischal A, Singh S, Dalal PK. Quality of life and disability in patients with Dhat syndrome: a cross-sectional study. Indian J Psychol Med. 2022;44(5):459–65. https://doi.org/10.1177/02537176221078422.

Singh G. Dhat syndrome revisited. Indian J Psychiatry. 1985;27(2):119–22.

Singh A, Tripathi A, Gupta B, Agarwal V. Pathways to care for Dhat (semen loss anxiety) syndrome: a study from North India. Int J Ment Health. 2016;45(4):253–61. https://doi.org/10.1080/00207411.2016.1238741.

Strong YN, Li A, White ME, Razzak AN, Anderson DJ, Kaye AD, Herron EW, Khater NP, Cornett EM, Urits I. Dhat syndrome: epidemiology, risk factors, comorbidities, diagnosis, treatment, and management. Health Psychol Res. 2022;10(4):38759. https://doi.org/10.52965/001c.38759.

Udina M, Foulon H, Valdés M, Bhattacharyya S, Martín-Santos R. Dhat syndrome: a systematic review. Psychosomatics. 2013;54(3):212–8. https://doi.org/10.1016/j.psym.2012.09.003.

World Health Organization, editor. International statistical classification of diseases and related health problems. 10th revision, 2nd ed. World Health Organization; 2004.

# Chapter 6
# Comorbidities Associated with Dhat Syndrome

**Adarsh Tripathi and Saumya Upadhyay**

## 6.1 Introduction

A little more than 50 years ago, the term "Dhat syndrome" was used in South Asia for the first time to describe the typical clinical manifestations of young male patients who attributed their numerous physical, psychological and often sexual symptoms to semen loss. It is not a discrete disorder but it is a culturally influenced manifestation of syndrome reported by patients who mention a variety of symptoms, including impotence, anxiety, fatigue, weakness, many bodily ailments, and sad mood after real or perceived semen loss (American Psychiatric Association 2013).

The defining characteristic is the absence of any discernible physiological impairment and the anxiety and distress caused by the secretion of dhat. Patients describe dhat as a white/translucent, sticky discharge per penis that patients observed while urinating, defecating, and during sexual stimulation which is often precum or semen discharge during nocturnal emission. Ideas concerning this substance are connected to the culturally informed concept of dhatu (semen), which is one of the seven vital physiological fluids that must remain in balance to preserve health, according to the Hindu medical system Ayurveda. According to a widely held belief, forty droplets of butter produce one drop of blood, and forty droplets of blood produce one drop of semen; as a result, losing semen causes weakness both physically and mentally. This is known as the "Dhat syndrome," a term coined by Wig in the 1960s (Dhat-semen). This misconception is very common, especially among young people, who refer to whitish discharge at the onset or the end of urine flow as "Dhat."

In comparison to the West, Southeast Asian countries particularly India, Pakistan, Bangladesh and Nepal has a far more common and more severe reaction to the dread of semen loss. The fear of losing semen and the physical and mental power

A. Tripathi (✉) · S. Upadhyay
Department of Psychiatry, King George's Medical University, Lucknow, Uttar Pradesh, India

© The Author(s), under exclusive license to Springer Nature Singapore Pte Ltd. 2024

S. K. Kar et al. (eds.), *Dhat Syndrome*,
https://doi.org/10.1007/978-981-99-8870-9_6

that goes along with it is frequently compared to the castration complex, but in reality, the fear is primarily one of losing semen and of wanting to keep the beloved object. The idea that semen originates from every region of the body and serves as the self's creator raises the possibility of an extraordinarily potent cathexis on the semen, which is almost synonymous with the ego.

Although fear of semen loss has been reported from other parts of the world also. Along with the improvement in education, changes in culture, and the evolution of modern medical science, other parts of the world largely got rid of this idea of potential negative consequences of semen loss (Sumathipala et al. 2004). However, Southeast Asian countries continue to report high prevalence of this disorder.

## 6.2 Epidemiology

It is the most typical known case of culture-bound syndrome. It is most frequently reported from the subcontinent of India. Patients with Dhat syndrome are usually young and on average 26 years old. Since the syndrome is characterised by a fear of losing one's semen, these patients are typically men, though a related phenomenon has been reported in women also and it is commonly known as Female Dhat syndrome.

The majority of Dhat syndrome patients were found to be unmarried, have less schooling than their controls, and belong to lower socioeconomic backgrounds. These characteristics were also reported by demographic data from first-time patients referred to a psychosexual clinic in India. Up to two-third of cases were from rural areas (Strong et al. 2022).

## 6.3 Comorbidity

Depression is the most common co-morbidity of Dhat syndrome with a prevalence range of 40–66%. In addition, anxiety problems are present in 21–38% of individuals. Up to 40% of individuals have somatoform and hypochondriacal illnesses. In a multicentric study, about 20% of the patients were found to have comorbid depressive disorder, and another 20% were diagnosed with comorbid anxiety and somatoform disorders. About 50% of the population had comorbid sexual dysfunctions. Slightly higher than 20% had a combination of comorbid depressive and anxiety disorders (Sumathipala et al. 2004). According to a study by Dhikav et al., which included 30 patients in a tertiary care hospital, ten of them (33.3%) experienced premature ejaculation, and two (6.6%) had erectile dysfunction (Dhikav et al. 2007). Phobia, stress reactions, compulsive disorders, body dysmorphic disorders, and delusional disorders are among other less frequent comorbidities. Common symptoms of Dhat syndrome and commonly reported comorbidities are detailed in Tables 6.1 and 6.2.

**Table 6.1** Common symptoms associated with Dhat syndrome (Grover et al. 2015a, b; Jhanjee et al. 2011; Udina et al. 2013)

| | |
|---|---|
| Somatic complaints | 1. Bodily aches and pains<br>2. Burning or discoloured micturition<br>3. Increased frequency of micturition<br>4. Difficulty in micturition<br>5. Hollowing of eyes<br>6. Loss of control over the body<br>7. Weight loss<br>8. Loss of appetite<br>9. Vertigo/dizziness<br>10. Swelling of the body<br>11. Abdominal distension<br>12. Bloating<br>13. Passage of stool during micturition |
| Anxiety complaints | 1. Anxiety<br>2. Dryness of mouth/throat<br>3. Palpitation<br>4. Muscle tension<br>5. Fear of losing vital components of the body<br>6. Trembling |
| Depressive complaints | 1. Weakness<br>2. Guilt<br>3. Lethargy<br>4. Disturbed sleep<br>5. Loss of interest<br>6. Loss of attention/concentration<br>7. Loss of memory<br>8. Suicidal ideation<br>9. Low self-esteem |
| Sexual complaints | 1. Distortion of the shape of the penis<br>2. Genital itching<br>3. Genital boils and ulcers<br>4. Fear of sexual activity<br>5. Loss of libido<br>6. Erectile dysfunction<br>7. Premature ejaculation<br>8. Impotence |

**Table 6.2** Comorbidity in Dhat syndrome (Deb and Balhara 2013; Grover et al. 2015a, b)

| Comorbidity in Dhat syndrome | |
|---|---|
| No comorbidity | 30% |
| Depressive disorder | 40–60% |
| Somatoform disorder | 40% |
| OCD | 1–5% |
| Comorbid sexual dysfunction | 45–55% |
| Erectile dysfunction | 20–25% |
| Premature ejaculation | 20–30 |
| Both sexual dysfunction and psychiatric disorder | 20% |

### *6.3.1 Dhat Syndrome and Depression*

#### 6.3.1.1 Predisposition

The substantial comorbidity between depression and sexual issues indicates that both disorders may have a common psychological etiology. According to Nobre's cognitive-emotional model of sexual dysfunctions (Quinta Gomes and Nobre 2021), etiological factors that have consistently been linked to depressive disorders such as neuroticism, high negative trait affect, and low positive trait affect have an integrated effect on sexual problems (Fig. 6.1; Clark and Watson 1991).

Greater concern over penile size in these patients may occur due to either physical preoccupation or low self-esteem consistent with a depressed disposition (Veale et al. 2016).

These patients may also experience guilt over erotic dreams, masturbation and nightfall, making this feeling predominant in the background of depressive disorder. Additionally, these patients have been found to have less formal education, which might have influenced them to accept the widely held cultural idea that semen loss causes psychological and physical symptoms. Instead of being a distinct clinical

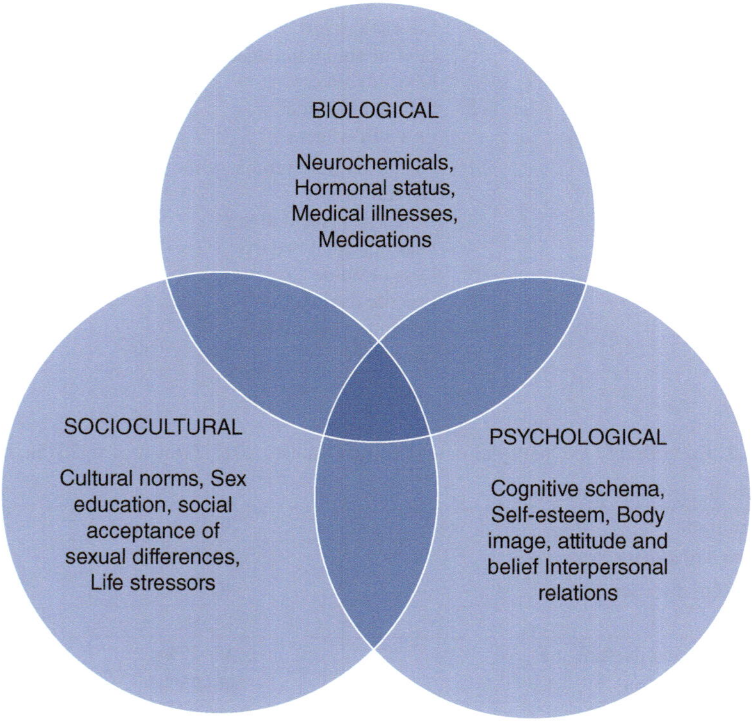


**Fig. 6.1** The biopsychosocial model of sexual response (Clark and Watson 1991)

entity, semen loss may be an explanatory model for their depressive symptoms (Dhikav et al. 2007).

Hence, Dhat syndrome could be a culturally-conditioned manifestation of a depressive disorder. Some evidence for this claim comes from earlier published research on the Dhat syndrome, which documents high rates of concomitant depression, ranging from 48 to 66%. Antidepressants seem to help Dhat syndrome patients, further pointing to a connection between both disorders. Studying the conceivable genetic link between Dhat syndrome and depression is one method of investigating this association (Grover et al. 2015a, b).

#### 6.3.1.2 Prevalence

With Dhat syndrome, the most frequent psychiatric diagnosis in terms of specific illnesses is depression. The prevalence of depression ranges from 40 to 66% (Deb and Balhara 2013). A retrospective study conducted at a tertiary care institution in India demonstrated that, compared to individuals without a family history of depressive spectrum disorders, patients with a family history of depressive disorders had a higher probability of developing depressive disorders or drug use disorders along with Dhat syndrome (Rajkumar and Bharadwaj 2014).

#### 6.3.1.3 Management

While psychological therapies, such as cognitive-behavioural therapy, are effective for treating lesser types of depression, moderate to severe depressive symptomatology needs a strategic approach combining psychiatric treatment (antidepressant medication) and psychological therapy. Additionally, the use of antidepressant drugs having little to no effect on sexual response in conjunction with psychotherapy is preferred to maximise treatment compliance and prevent early treatment cessation.

**Psychoeducation:** A helpful technique includes listening with empathy, a non-confrontational style, assurance and disbelief correction, as well as the use of anti-depressant medications.

The standardized treatment package for single males presenting with Dhat syndrome mainly includes sex education and relaxation exercises (Grover et al. 2016). In Dhat, sexual education primarily focuses on the anatomy and physiology of sexual organs as well as how they operate about things like masturbation, semen, nocturnal emissions, and the genitourinary system, among other things. To promote objective evidence and to help the patient master anxiety, relaxation treatment involves Jacobson's Progressive Muscular Relaxation Technique mixed with Bio-feedback, which should be practised routinely 2–3 times/day, especially after therapy sessions are ended.

According to a study conducted on 40 male Dhat syndrome patients, those who received supportive psychotherapy (with an emphasis on relaxation and psychoeducation) in addition to Ayurvedic therapy scored significantly lower on the Hamilton Depression Rating Scale (HAM-D) after 1 month than those who received only Ayurvedic therapy.

**Mindfulness**: The patient's capacity to focus and concentrate during mindfulness activities may be hampered by the well-known detrimental effects of depression on the cognitive system. However, it can be an important way to deal with preoccupations associated with low mood in Dhat syndrome.

**Cognitive restructuring:** In the Cognitive Behavioural Therapy (CBT) module, the emphasis is placed on the emotional and interpersonal components of sexuality, in addition to the different cognitive distortions that are treated. Issues with performance anxiety address the entwined masculinity and sexual power schema. In cases of sexual dysfunction, other strategies are taught, such as Jacobson's Progressive Muscle Relaxation (JPMR), imaginal desensitisation, masturbation as homework to comprehend the harmless loss of semen, Kegel's exercises, and squeeze and start-stop procedures (Salam et al. 2012).

Selective serotonin reuptake inhibitors help to treat comorbid depression and Dhat syndrome (Dhikav et al. 2007). There is, however, no established consensus or guideline. The patient's willingness to get therapy and the treating psychiatrist's assessment of the patient's symptoms play a significant role in the clinical decision. Using psychotropic medications mainly SSRIs along with psychological interventions may help in retaining patients for the long-term in treatment hence improving outcome and prognosis. However, one should exercise appropriate caution when prescribing pharmaceuticals to avoid aggravating pre-existing issues with the medication's frequent negative effects. SSRIs may have sexual side effects which may exacerbate already existing sexual dysfunctions related to comorbidities of Dhat syndrome. Fluoxetine and Sertraline, two SSRIs with early activating effects, may make anxiety and restlessness worse. Potent long-acting benzodiazepines can cause sedation, daytime sleepiness, exacerbation of fatigue, giddiness, and cognitive problems (Grover et al. 2015a, b; Avasthi and Gupta 1997).

## *6.3.2 Dhat Syndrome and Somatoform Disorders*

### 6.3.2.1 Predisposition

Dhat syndrome can also be viewed as an abnormal disease behaviour that manifests semen loss in an increased type of somatization and heightened emotional reactivity. Patients with Dhat syndrome experience a great deal of stress. When stress is present, the onset of stress symptoms is accelerated. People who have Dhat syndrome see their semen discharge pathologically and as a result, give it undue weight.

They endure stress if they lose semen because it is not seen as natural in their culture. Due to this pathologic way of perceiving, the stress response becomes conditioned with semen loss, and the vicious cycle continues. The initial stress experience is compounded over time in this conditioning process, which causes the psychosomatic symptoms of Dhat syndrome to be exaggerated (Kar and Sarkar 2015).

Dhat syndrome symptoms include fatigue frequently (Bhatia and Malik 1991). As functional somatic syndromes, disorders with exhaustion as their primary symptom are frequently categorised together. The fundamental cognitive model put out to explain these disorders is based on abnormal illness behaviour, somatosensory amplification, and misattribution.

The socio-somatic framework has been merged with societal and cultural aspects to explain dhat syndrome as a functional somatic syndrome (Kirmayer and Young 1998).

The urogenital system is likely to be the subject of worry in societies where discussing sexual problems openly is frowned upon and there are worries about masturbating.

When under stress, those who are prone to exaggerating somatic symptoms and health worries may draw attention to physiological changes such as discoloured urine and fatigue and mistakenly attribute them to semen loss in light of generally held health beliefs. Then, peer groups, other lay sources, and local practitioners who follow related approaches may corroborate or even enhance these ideas.

#### 6.3.2.2 Prevalence

The prevalence of somatoform and hypochondriacal disorders in Dhat syndrome patients has been reported to be around 40% (Deb and Balhara 2013).

#### 6.3.2.3 Management

Therapists must emphasize that, even though the physical source of their problem has not been identified and it is thought that the symptoms' root cause is psychological. Physicians acknowledge the distress and impairments caused by symptoms and reassure the patients that symptoms are fake, false or not genuine. Usually, it takes the patient a long time to accept that his or her problems are psychological in nature.

However, psychoeducation remains the key along with pharmacological management as for somatoform disorder preferably in the form of SNRIs or tricyclic antidepressants may be beneficial.

### *6.3.3 Dhat Syndrome and Obsessive-Compulsive Disorders*

#### 6.3.3.1 Predisposition

The factors contributing to both could include a vulnerability to anxiety disorders, cultural beliefs and attitudes toward bodily functions, and individual variations in symptom expression and coping mechanisms. Obsessive thoughts about semen and the negative effects of its discharge are typical of Dhat syndrome in this case. The obsessional quality may make the patient anxious enough to force him to engage in repetitive checking behaviours that are sufficient for an OCD diagnosis.

#### 6.3.3.2 Prevalence

It is important to note that the prevalence rates of Dhat syndrome and OCD can vary widely across different cultural and geographical contexts. However, OCD with Dhat syndrome is not a commonly found diagnosis. The comorbid association between OCD and dhat syndrome has been reported to be low (Grover et al. 2015a).

#### 6.3.3.3 Management

In the co-occurrence of OCD and Dhat syndrome on an individual basis, considering the unique circumstances of each person is necessary.

SSRI's would improve the obsessional thoughts, compulsive acts as well as concerns related to Dhat syndrome. Psychoeducation regarding dysfunctional beliefs is a must. Cognitive behavioural therapy is helpful (Ghosh and Chowdhury 2020). Other behavioural techniques like exposure response prevention do not have enough supporting evidence but may be tried considering the individual's clinical profile.

### *6.3.4 Dhat Syndrome and Psychosexual Disorders*

#### 6.3.4.1 Predisposition

One of the most prevalent illnesses, sexual dysfunctions, are characterized by alterations in the pathophysiology of the sexual response cycle or in sexual desire that prevent an individual or a couple from experiencing sexual satisfaction. Relationships with others or a person's quality of life are negatively impacted by sexual dysfunction (Pal et al. 2017).

Disorders like premature ejaculation and erectile dysfunction strongly affect male self-esteem and may lead to the development of neurotic disorders which, in the background of sexual dysfunction, gives way to a preoccupation with the passage of semen. Alternatively, preoccupation and misconceptions regarding semen loss along with the associated anxiety may influence a person's sexual performance and ability to perceive pleasure.

#### 6.3.4.2 Prevalence

One of the frequent causes people visit psychosexual clinics is the Dhat syndrome. It makes up about 18% of all patients seeking therapy for psychosexual problems (Verma et al. 2013). A statewide multicentric study carried out in India revealed that Dhat syndrome was identified in one-third of the patients without any form of concomitant psychiatric condition or sexual dysfunction. Only about 40% of patients had co-occurring psychiatric problems and 50% had co-occurring sexual dysfunction overall. The most prevalent comorbid sexual dysfunction is premature ejaculation, which is observed in around one-third of patients.

Erectile dysfunction, which affects around a fifth of patients, is the second most common. Dhat syndrome can have psychosexual dysfunction or not. Researchers have divided the Dhat syndrome into three subgroups based on the comorbidity: the Dhat syndrome alone, the Dhat syndrome with anxiety and depressive symptoms, and the Dhat syndrome with sexual dysfunction (Udina et al. 2013).

#### 6.3.4.3 Management

Sexual education, relaxation exercises and clarifying of sexual myths are important, in addition, homework assignments in the form of genital and non-genital sensate focus have been found beneficial. Pharmacological treatment consists of medications, constriction rings, vacuum constriction devices, intra-cavernosal injections, intra-urethral medication devices, penile prostheses and reconstructive surgery. However, pharmacological methods should be instituted carefully after thorough review and examination. In view of the management, it is fruitful to pay attention to whether the sexual dysfunction developed secondary to Dhat syndrome, or if it was the primary condition.

### *6.3.5 Dhat Syndrome and Schizophrenia*

#### 6.3.5.1 Predisposition

Dhat syndrome is sometimes referred to as a prodrome of schizophrenia in case reports. Wide range of symptoms, including frequent somatic symptoms, have been observed in the schizophrenia prodrome. Before developing into schizophrenia, the prodromal symptoms may persist for weeks to years. The transition from prodrome to schizophrenia is the result of a complex interplay of vulnerability factors (neurodevelopmental and psychosocial), stress-gene interaction, and the body's defence mechanism.

Patients frequently exhibit a variety of vague physical symptoms, anxiety, and anguish, which they blame on semen loss. Schizophrenia is one of many mental illnesses for which stress is a known risk factor. Stress, which can begin as early as the prodromal stage of schizophrenia, may cause hypothalamo-pituitary-adrenal axis disruption. Through epigenetic pathways, stress can interfere with the regular operation of the psyche. The transition from the prodromal phase to schizophrenia is mediated by several stress-related characteristics, including early life traumas, a malfunctioning stress response, and increased stress sensitivity. Stress brought on by semen loss may be a key factor in these patients' change (Kar et al. 2016).

#### 6.3.5.2 Prevalence

The prevalence of Dhat syndrome with schizophrenia has not been studied adequately, likely due to prodromal symptoms being largely unattended. Understanding the cultural concepts of distress may be helpful for the clinician in understanding various symptom domains of the prodromal phase of schizophrenia.

#### 6.3.5.3 Management

Psychoeducation and biological explanations may be delivered over multiple sessions, along with treatment with appropriate dose-adjusted antipsychotics.

## 6.4 Current Status and Research Gaps in the Literature Regarding Comorbidity

The prevalence data of comorbidities in Dhat syndrome are sufficiently reported. However, the nature, bidirectional interaction, impact on the course, prognosis and management strategies are yet to be scientifically studied. Etiopathological evidence of causative factors in psychiatric disorders are difficult to ascertain. However, in the case of Dhat syndrome and its associated comorbidities, the debate has just begun about the relative contribution of various factors that can contribute to the causation of these illnesses.

## 6.5 Conclusion

Comorbidities in Dhat syndrome are common and significantly impact levels of disability, quality of life and functioning in comparison to subjects who only have Dhat syndrome (Shahi et al. 2022). The course and prognosis of the illness are considerably influenced by the clinician should consider possibility of comorbidities in each case of Dhat syndrome. Strategies during clinical assessment, application of clinical interventions and monitoring should be tailored according to the additional comorbidities. Management of dhat syndrome and comorbidities is conducted simultaneously. There is a need to continue research on patterns, characteristics and mutual impact of dhat syndrome and comorbidities on each other.

## References

American Psychiatric Association. Diagnostic and statistical manual of mental and behavioural disorders DSM-V. Washington: American Psychiatric Association; 2013.

Avasthi A, Gupta N. Manual for standardized management of single males with sexual disorders. Chandigarh: Marital and Psychosexual Clinic; 1997.

Bhatia MS, Malik SC. Dhat syndrome—a useful diagnostic entity in Indian culture. Br J Psychiatry. 1991;159(5):691–5.

Clark LA, Watson D. Tripartite model of anxiety and depression: psychometric evidence and taxonomic implications. J Abnorm Psychol. 1991;100(3):316.

Deb KS, Balhara YPS. Dhat syndrome: a review of the world literature. Indian J Psychol Med. 2013;35(4):326–31.

Dhikav V, Aggarwal N, Anand KS. Is Dhat syndrome, a culturally appropriate manifestation of depression? Med Hypotheses. 2007;69(3):698.

Ghosh S, Chowdhury AN. A case of two culture-bound syndromes (Koro and Dhat syndrome) coexisting with obsessive-compulsive disorder. Indian J Psychiatry. 2020;62(2):221–2.

Grover S, Avasthi A, Gupta S, Dan A, Neogi R, Behere PB, et al. Comorbidity in patients with Dhat syndrome: a nationwide multicentric study. J Sex Med. 2015a;12(6):1398–401.

Grover S, Gupta S, Avasthi A. Psychological correlates and psychiatric morbidity in patients with Dhat syndrome. Indian J Psychiatry. 2015b;57(3):255.

Grover S, Gupta S, Avasthi A. A follow-up study of patients with Dhat syndrome: Treatment pattern, outcome, and reasons for dropout from treatment. Indian J Psychiatry. 2016;58(1):49–56. https://doi.org/10.4103/0019-5545.174373.

Jhanjee A, Bhatia MS, Kumar P. A study on comorbidities, knowledge and attitudes among patients of Dhat syndrome. Eur Psychiatry. 2011;26(S2):460.

Kar SK, Sarkar S. Dhat syndrome: evolution of concept, current understanding, and need of an integrated approach. J Hum Reprod Sci. 2015;8(3):130.

Kar SK, Shahi MK, Tripathi A. Dhat syndrome as the prodrome of schizophrenia: understanding the cultural distress. Asian J Psychiatr. 2016;25:203–4.

Kirmayer LJ, Young A. Culture and somatization: clinical, epidemiological, and ethnographic perspectives. Psychosom Med. 1998;60(4):420–30.

Pal A, Mallik N, Acharya R, Mondal DK. Epidemiology of patients attending a special clinic on sexual dysfunction from Eastern India: a retrospective data review. Med J Dr. DY Patil Univ. 2017;10(6):542–7.

Quinta Gomes AL, Nobre PJ. Depressive disorders. In: Psychiatry and sexual medicine: a comprehensive guide for clinical practitioners. 2021. p. 235–48.

Rajkumar RP, Bharadwaj B. Dhat syndrome: evidence for a depressive spectrum subtype. Asian J Psychiatr. 2014;9:57–60.

Salam KA, Sharma MP, Prakash O. Development of cognitive-behavioral therapy intervention for patients with Dhat syndrome. Indian J Psychiatry. 2012;54(4):367.

Shahi MK, Tripathi A, Singh A, Kar SK, Nischal A, Singh S, Dalal PK. Quality of life and disability in patients with dhat syndrome: a cross-sectional study. Indian J Psychol Med. 2022;44(5):459–65.

Strong YN, Li A, White ME, Razzak AN, Anderson DJ, Kaye AD, et al. Dhat syndrome: epidemiology, risk factors, comorbidities, diagnosis, treatment, and management. Health Psychol Res. 2022;10(4):38759.

Sumathipala A, Siribaddana SH, Bhugra D. Culture-bound syndromes: the story of dhat syndrome. Br J Psychiatry. 2004;184(3):200–9.

Veale D, Miles S, Read J, Bramley S, Troglia A, Carmona L, Fiorito C, Wells H, Wylie K, Muir G. Relationship between self-discrepancy and worries about penis size in men with body dysmorphic disorder. Body Image. 2016;17:48–56. https://doi.org/10.1016/j.bodyim.2016.02.004.

Udina M, Foulon H, Valdés M, Bhattacharyya S, Martín-Santos R. Dhat syndrome: a systematic review. Psychosomatics. 2013;54(3):212–8.

Verma R, Mina S, Ul-Hassan S, Balhara YPS. A descriptive analysis of patients presenting to psychosexual clinic at a tertiary care center. Indian J Psychol Med. 2013;35(3):241–7.

Winokur G, Coryell W. Familial subtypes of unipolar depression: a prospective study of familial pure depressive disease compared to depression spectrum disease. Biol Psychiatry. 1992;32(11):1012–8.

# Chapter 7
# Care-Seeking, Pathway to Care and Disease Burden in Dhat Syndrome

**Amit Singh**

## 7.1 Introduction

Dhat syndrome is a common presentation in psychosexual clinics in South Asian countries (Kendurkar et al. 2008). It has roots in the culturally embedded beliefs of the preciousness of semen, which is perceived as a vital life force associated with masculinity and virility (Prakash et al. 2014). The conservation of semen is highly emphasized in ancient Indian medicinal texts, where the loss of semen is equated with the loss of masculinity, power, and fertility, and leads to a decline in physical and psychological strength and even premature death. Typically, in Dhat syndrome there is an excessive preoccupation with semen loss during masturbation, nocturnal emissions, micturition, or defecation. Beliefs such as premarital sexual intercourse and excessive indulgence in sexual activities causing 'semen loss' is also common. Thus, among people from these cultural backgrounds, any perceived excessive or involuntary loss of semen can instil an intense fear of losing virility and other adverse consequences (Prakash et al. 2014). This fear often causes significant distress, contributing to social, emotional, and sexual difficulties among affected individuals.

Impairment caused to the affected individuals due to Dhat syndrome may be very high, especially in the presence of co-occurring disorders (Shahi et al. 2022). However, the help-seeking and pathway to care are highly diverse, which even impacts the course and outcomes of the disorder per se. Thus, Dhat syndrome presents unique challenges to both, the affected individuals and the healthcare providers. This article explores the complexities surrounding help-seeking behaviours, pathways to care, and the burden this disorder imposes on the affected individuals and society. A better understanding of which is important in improving diagnosis, treatment plans, and the overall well-being of affected individuals.

A. Singh (✉)
Department of Psychiatry, King George's Medical University, Lucknow, India

© The Author(s), under exclusive license to Springer Nature Singapore Pte Ltd. 2024
S. K. Kar et al. (eds.), *Dhat Syndrome*,
https://doi.org/10.1007/978-981-99-8870-9_7

## 7.2 Pathways to Care

Pathways to care refers to the series of interactions with people and organizations brought on by the efforts of patients and their concerned ones to reach out for help (Rogler and Cortes 1993). Goldberg and Huxley in the 1980s proposed the model of 'pathway' to psychiatric care to provide a theoretical framework for the processes individuals go through when seeking mental health care (Goldberg and Huxley 2001). The model consisted of five service levels and four variably permeable filters, through which a person in the community has to pass through to avail health care from a mental health specialist. The filters imply key determinants that limit a fraction of individuals from moving to the next level. It includes the decision to seek help, identification of the disorder by general practitioners, and subsequent referrals. However, it should be noted that the model in its original form is not universally applicable. Over the years, deviations have been observed concerning various disorders and geographical contexts, leading to suggestions for modification (Sorketti et al. 2013). For instance, in many countries where Dhat syndrome is common, the healthcare system is not hierarchical and people can bypass various levels and filters to directly consult mental health specialists without any referral from a general practitioner. Also, the pathway to care in Dhat syndrome may not follow a linear progression and can involve multiple iterations between different levels. Nevertheless, the key concepts emerging from the model are useful in understanding the factors that influence help-seeking behaviour for mental health issues including Dhat syndrome. It also highlights the importance of recognizing mental health problems, reducing stigma, and facilitating timely access to specialist care and underscores the role of various stakeholders, including individuals, their social network, and healthcare providers, in supporting individuals through the help-seeking process and promoting positive mental health outcomes.

### *7.2.1 Care-Seeking*

In Dhat syndrome the perceived loss of semen concerns affected individuals. Surrounding fears regarding the loss of potency or virility and adverse consequences to health compels them to seek clarifications, medical explanations, and potential remedies for their symptoms (Singh et al. 2016). A variety of physical symptoms such as fatigue, weakness, back pain, genital discomfort, and urinary problems, and psychiatric issues such as depression and anxiety may also be present. Besides, the commonly co-occurring psychosexual disorders such as erectile dysfunction and premature ejaculation may be concerning to the individuals (Singh 1985). The distress and functional impairment due to these symptoms can interfere with daily activities, work, and relationships and impact the overall quality of life, motivating them to seek medical attention. The healthcare-seeking behaviour is influenced by a variety of factors, including cultural norms, stigma, awareness levels, and access to healthcare services.

#### 7.2.1.1 Cultural Factors

Cultural norms and values play a vital role in shaping healthcare-seeking behaviour in Dhat syndrome, especially in South Asian countries such as India, Pakistan, Bangladesh, Nepal, and Sri Lanka (Kar et al. 2021). In these geographies, sexual illnesses are often met with strong aversion and societal disdain. Topics related to sex and sexual health are often considered taboo, making it difficult for individuals to seek timely medical assistance for psychosexual disorders. Besides, Dhat syndrome is more common among men belonging to rural backgrounds where conservative societal attitudes towards sex, gender roles, and relationships may hinder them from seeking help, fearing social judgment and negative consequences on their reputation or family honor (Khan 2005).

#### 7.2.1.2 Stigma and Shame

Psychosexual disorders, in general, are associated with higher stigma and shame. Dhat syndrome is no exception. In South Asian societies, the presence of deep-rooted stigma surrounding sexual illnesses which are perceived as immoral, dirty, or shameful, contributes to this abhorrence (Chakraborty and Thakurata 2013). Besides, stigma and discrimination are also present for mental health and psychosexual disorders. Affected individuals are likely to experience social isolation, ridicule, and even discrimination in various aspects of their lives. Fear of being stigmatized or labeled as "sexually weak" or "mentally ill" leads to silence and secrecy, often preventing individuals from seeking professional help (Khan 2005). This exacerbates their distress and hinders timely and appropriate healthcare and support.

#### 7.2.1.3 Awareness and Education

Limited awareness and knowledge of sexual disorders contribute to the challenges in healthcare-seeking behaviour (Grover et al. 2015, 2016a). Regarding Dhat syndrome, inadequate sexual education and a dearth of public discourse around psychosexual health perpetuate the existing knowledge gaps. Affected individuals often lack knowledge about the nature of the problem, management approach as well as the care provider to consult for help. This gives rise to a variety of misconceptions and misinformation and hinders individuals from recognizing their symptoms and seeking care from specialists. Also common is the false recognition of otherwise normal bodily phenomena and human behaviours such as nocturnal emissions and masturbation as abnormal, causing distress and self-blame (Grover et al. 2016a).

Dhat syndrome is more common in people who are uneducated or have less formal education. People when reach out to quacks or unqualified medical practitioners for help in this regard are often misguided into believing that they are suffering from a severe medical condition, reinforcing their false beliefs (Ranjith and Mohan 2006).

#### 7.2.1.4 Social Factors

The support of family members and the community plays a vital role in influencing care-seeking decisions in psychiatric disorders. Family, peers, and social networks are the initial sources of information about Dhat syndrome and their recommendations influence the choice of care-seeking options (Chadda et al. 2001; Singh et al. 2016; Acharjee and Mullick 2021). Shoib et al. (2018) reported that patients received knowledge regarding Dhat syndrome from friends and colleagues in 46% of cases, relatives provided knowledge in 18% of cases, mass media, magazines and posters accounted for 22% of cases, while quacks provided information in 14% of cases (Shoib et al. 2018). Also, societal attitudes and norms largely impact the help-seeking behaviour.

#### 7.2.1.5 Healthcare System-Related Factors

Access to specialized healthcare services for psychosexual diseases is often limited in South Asian countries. Many individuals in rural or marginalized communities have limited access to healthcare facilities and face financial constraints that prevent them from seeking medical assistance (Chadda et al. 2001). The shortage of mental health professionals with expertise in psychiatric disorders and Dhat syndrome management further restricts access to appropriate care. Besides, general physicians are often not trained in managing culture-bound syndromes like Dhat syndrome, especially in the aspects of psychoeducation and sex therapy which are inadequately integrated into mainstream healthcare systems. Thus, referral practices, as well as collaboration and coordination among healthcare providers are important determinants in care-seeking pathways. Also, individual perceptions of the effectiveness of healthcare interventions influence care-seeking decisions.

### *7.2.2 Healthcare Providers (Sources of Care Seeking)*

Patients with Dhat syndrome may consult various individuals or professionals for help, depending on cultural beliefs, accessibility, and personal preferences.

#### 7.2.2.1 Initial Self-Help or Informal Support

Some individuals may initially try to manage their symptoms on their own or seek advice from family, friends, or other trusted individuals in their social circle before approaching healthcare professionals (Shoib et al. 2018). This may involve traditional remedies, over-the-counter medications, lifestyle changes, or advice from others who have experienced similar symptoms. This informal support can provide reassurance or reinforce cultural beliefs about Dhat syndrome. Currently, people also turn to online resources to seek information. However, not all information available on these platforms is correct and may conversely exacerbate their worries.

#### 7.2.2.2 Traditional Healers and Unqualified 'Sex Specialists'

In South Asian cultures, individuals with Dhat syndrome often consult unqualified alternative medicine practitioners (such as *vaids*, *hakims*, and '*sex specialists*'), faith healers, or religious leaders (such as priests, imams, or gurus) who are believed to have expertise in treating such conditions. These practitioners may employ counselling, culturally specific remedies, herbs, or alternative therapies to address the perceived loss of vital fluid and associated distress (Prakash et al. 2018). However, because of a poor understanding of the biological underpinnings of the phenomenon, there is a high likelihood of them providing inadequate or inappropriate information about the phenomenon.

#### 7.2.2.3 General Physicians and Qualified Alternative Medicine Practitioners

When the symptoms persist or worsen, patients may visit general practitioners or primary care physicians who happen to be allopathic doctors or qualified alternative medicine practitioners (such as Ayurveda, Unani, Siddha, Homeopathy, and Naturopathy). Primary care physicians usually inquire about symptoms, conduct general physical examinations, and get done relevant laboratory investigations to rule out any underlying medical conditions that could be contributing to the symptoms. The initial advice or treatment provided by them often helps affected individuals. However, due to the lack of expertise in managing Dhat syndrome, resource constraints, and high illness severity, many patients fail to achieve complete relief.

#### 7.2.2.4 Specialist Care

In some cases, people themselves consult or are referred by primary care physicians/general practitioners to specialists such as psychiatrists, dermatologists, or urologists for further evaluation and management. This step is important to rule out any underlying medical conditions that may contribute to the symptoms and to address the psychological aspects of Dhat syndrome. Specialists can provide more targeted evaluations, interventions, and management strategies tailored to Dhat syndrome. Given the significant psychological distress associated with Dhat syndrome, the mental health professionals, such as psychiatrists or psychologists, play a crucial role in the care of Dhat syndrome patients. They conduct a thorough psychological assessment to understand the patient's beliefs, cultural context, and psychological distress. Appropriate interventions may include psychoeducation, supportive counseling, psychotherapy including cognitive-behavioural therapy (CBT), or pharmacotherapy for comorbid conditions such as anxiety or depression (Kar and Sarkar 2015).

Behere and Natraj (1984) reported the consultation pattern in research comprising 50 Dhat syndrome outpatients. Their findings revealed that unqualified "sex specialists" were the initial healthcare providers in the majority of cases (50%). It was followed by skin and venereal disease specialists (30%), and general practitioners (20%) (Behere and Natraj 1984). According to De Silva and Dissanayake (1989), almost all of their patients sought prior treatment from Ayurvedic doctors. About 10% of the patients sought treatment from homoeopathic practitioners or had folk remedies. Around a third of the patients also consulted allopathic practitioners at some stage (De Silva and Dissanayake 1989). According to a study conducted in Pakistan, approximately half of the patients sought the assistance of *hakims*, followed by homeopaths (23.6%) and general physicians (18.6%). Only a small percentage (2.3%) of patients sought help from psychiatrists and psychologists (Khan 2005). According to Grover et al. (2016a, b), the most frequent initial contact was with qualified alternative medicine (mainly Ayurvedic) practitioners (36.2%), followed by assistance from friends or family (31.9%), allopathic physicians (23.4%) including general physicians, urologists, and surgeons, and conventional faith healers or chemists (8.5%) (Grover et al. 2016b). Similarly, Singh et al. (2016) found that for initial help 49.1% of the patients turned to unqualified healthcare practitioners, 25% to general physicians, 18.2% to qualified practitioners of alternative medicine, and less than 10% to psychiatrists. Further, during the pathway to specialist care, more than 60% of patients consult unqualified practitioners or general physicians at some stage, whereas around half of patients sought the advice of practitioners of alternative medicine (Singh et al. 2016).

Hence, it is evident that patients with Dhat syndrome predominantly seek initial consultations with unqualified practitioners or alternative medicine practitioners along their pathway to care. This help-seeking pattern is largely shaped by prevailing cultural beliefs surrounding the Dhat syndrome. A survey conducted in an urban slum in India with 1344 male participants found that a sizable majority (42%) think that Ayurveda, Homoeopathy, and Unani systems of medicine offer effective treatments for semen loss. It also revealed a poor understanding of people about Dhat syndrome (Verma et al. 2003). Besides, it is common among faith healers and unqualified traditional practitioners to advertise treatment for sexual issues and even make guarantees of complete recovery from Dhat syndrome. Thus, patients are often drawn to them to seek help for Dhat syndrome in conservative societies. Additional significant factor contributing to this trend is that unqualified traditional practitioners are readily available, simple to reach, and affordable; whereas, there is a shortage of mental health specialists in the region.

### 7.2.3 *Help-Seeking Delay*

The Dhat syndrome causes considerable distress and morbidity. However, many patients delay disclosing their problems to others or seeking help. Also, the dilemma of whom and when to consult results in wasted time. Furthermore, the understanding of family, friends, and acquaintances regarding normal sex physiology and Dhat syndrome is often unsatisfactory; thus, they fail to provide the patient with the necessary support and help in finding appropriate solutions. As a result, there is a significant delay in patients seeking help.

A study found that the average illness duration before the first consultation with a care provider was 1.85(±2.14) years. There was an additional delay of 4.63(±5.35) years between the first care provider consultation and consultation with a psychiatrist, indicating a substantial amount of time wasted in the process of seeking appropriate healthcare (Singh et al. 2016). Studies specifically assessing the pathway of care in Dhat syndrome reported approximately 6 years of delay before consulting a psychiatrist/mental health care facility (Grover et al. 2016b; Singh et al. 2016). Though there is a high variation in the duration, between months and decades, before consulting a psychiatrist/mental health care facility (Grover et al. 2016a, b; Singh et al. 2016).

It is surmisable that the intermediate care providers do not provide adequate information to the patients regarding the availability of specialist care for Dhat syndrome. This is apparent from the lower proportion of referrals made by them for psychiatric consultations (Singh et al. 2016). Also, the traditional healers and unqualified sex specialists may be reinforcing myths and misconceptions related to Dhat syndrome intensifying the fear and anxiety among patients (Kar and Varma 1978). As a result, patients seek help from multiple healthcare providers and make repeated visits, leading to a significant loss of time and resources without experiencing substantial symptom relief. Grover et al. (2016a, b) noticed a gradual decline in preference for visiting indigenous practitioners at each stage (Grover et al. 2016b).

### 7.2.4 *Referral Pattern of Patients*

Patients seeking information about 'Dhat Syndrome' are exposed to various sources that encourage them to consult healthcare providers for assistance. In many cases, patients independently seek help and approach caregivers based on billboards, advertisements, and hearsay information. This self-referred group constitutes the majority (approximately 58%) of patients who initially consult a healthcare provider for assistance (Singh et al. 2016). Grover et al. (2015) also reported that individuals initially seek guidance and help from friends, colleagues, elders, relatives, or unqualified healthcare providers, as well as through unscientific sex literature, rather than qualified practitioners of modern medicine (Grover et al. 2015). Additionally, family members, friends, co-workers, neighbors, and relatives play a significant role as sources of referral. On average, patients consult about three caregivers before reaching out to a psychiatrist (Grover et al. 2016b). According to Singh et al. (2016), over 50% of patients consulted three or more care providers before finally consulting a psychiatrist. The study found that even late in the course of illness, the decision to consult psychiatrists was made either based on accumulating self-knowledge (40.0%) or the suggestions of relatives and other social contacts (40%). The knowledge about the nature of the problem among various care providers is also likely to be poor, as indicated by the referral patterns to psychiatrists (Prakash et al. 2018). Only 20% of referrals were made by other healthcare providers (Singh et al. 2016). However, there may be wide geographical variation in the referral pattern to psychiatrists. Shoib et al. (2018), reported that around 80% of their patients were referred by allopathic practitioners (46% by dermatologists, 18% by physicians, and 16% by surgeons). 14% of patients directly came to the psychiatrist (Shoib et al. 2018).

To overcome the challenges in pathways of care, it is essential to educate and increase awareness among affected and vulnerable individuals, healthcare professionals, and the community about Dhat syndrome. Awareness generation efforts should also focus on destigmatizing mental health and promoting open discussions about psychosexual disorders (Kar and Singh 2016). This can lead to early recognition of Dhat syndrome and appropriate referrals for specialized care. Engaging community leaders and influential figures can also help in normalizing discussions about sexual health and encouraging individuals to seek healthcare services without fear or judgment.

Another important issue that needs to be addressed is that of accessibility and affordability of services. Access to quality healthcare services is a significant barrier to healthcare-seeking in many South Asian countries. Improving infrastructure, expanding healthcare services, and training healthcare providers are essential steps toward ensuring access to comprehensive sexual health services for all segments of society (Kar and Sarkar 2015). Telemedicine and online platforms can also play a significant role in reaching individuals in remote areas and providing them with expert guidance and support.

Also, culturally sensitive approaches within healthcare systems can help address stigma, enhance communication, and improve treatment outcomes. Thus, healthcare providers should approach patients with cultural sensitivity, acknowledging their beliefs, and avoiding stigmatization or invalidation.

Encouraging collaboration between traditional healers, primary care physicians, and mental health professionals can lead to better integration of traditional practices with evidence-based treatments (Kar and Sarkar 2015). Besides, the sources spreading misinformation about Dhat syndrome in public should be controlled. The healthcare for Dhat syndrome patients should be comprehensive, encompassing medical, psychological, and cultural dimensions, and it should be tailored to meet the unique needs and beliefs of the individual.

## 7.3 Burden Associated with Dhat Syndrome

The healthcare burden associated with Dhat syndrome is multifaceted and can have significant implications for both individuals and healthcare systems. Being largely a culture-bound syndrome, it may not be widely recognized or understood outside of specific cultural contexts, particularly in Western healthcare systems. Besides, the symptoms may overlap with other medical or psychological conditions. As a result, there may be delays in diagnosis. Ensuing multiple consultations and unnecessary investigations strain healthcare resources, increases healthcare costs, and creates a burden on the healthcare system (Arafat and Ahmed 2017). De Silva and Dissanayake (1989) reported patients spend manifold their monthly income over treatment during the pathway to care (De Silva and Dissanayake 1989).

Dhat syndrome is commonly associated with comorbid psychiatric conditions such as depression, anxiety, somatoform disorder, and psychosexual disorders (Grover et al. 2015). Managing these conditions require additional resources and specialized treatments, increasing the burden on mental healthcare systems. A study evaluating the quality of life and disability in patients with Dhat syndrome found the patients to have a poor quality of life compared to healthy controls. Besides, the presence of comorbid disorders resulted in significantly lower scores on quality of life and disability (Shahi et al. 2022). There may be a bidirectional relationship between quality of life and comorbidities. The distress leading to poor quality of life in Dhat syndrome may give rise to comorbidities and the presence of comorbidities substantially contribute to the quality of life worsening. Cultural barriers and stigma surrounding Dhat syndrome also delay help-seeking. This leads to the patients presenting to the healthcare system when the condition becomes more severe.

The distress associated with Dhat syndrome can significantly impact the quality of life and well-being of individuals. This can lead to impaired social functioning, occupational performance, and reduced productivity. Moreover, it may adversely impact sexual relationships leading to sexual dissatisfaction marital conflicts, and marital discord.

## 7.4 Conclusion

Pathways of care in Dhat syndrome are multifaceted, influenced by cultural beliefs, social factors, and the availability of healthcare resources. Patients initially seek assistance from various sources before eventually turning to formal healthcare. However, this process of searching for the appropriate care provider often results in substantial wastage of resources and increased healthcare burden. Thus, it is crucial to enhance awareness among vulnerable populations, address social stigma, establish an efficient and effective referral mechanism to expedite access to specialist care, and improve collaboration and cultural competence among healthcare professionals to reduce the overall healthcare burden associated with Dhat syndrome.

## References


Acharjee P, Mullick MSI. The pattern of help-seeking behavior among patients with sexual dysfunctions attending in psychiatry outpatient department in a tertiary care Hospital of Bangladesh. Sex Med. 2021;9:100381. https://doi.org/10.1016/j.esxm.2021.100381.

Arafat SMY, Ahmed S. Burden of misconception in sexual health care setting: a cross-sectional investigation among the patients attending a psychiatric sex clinic of Bangladesh. Psychiatry J. 2017;2017:9827083. https://doi.org/10.1155/2017/9827083.

Behere PB, Natraj GS. Dhat syndrome: the phenomenology of a culture bound sex neurosis of the orient. Indian J Psychiatry. 1984;26:76–8.

Chadda RK, Agarwal V, Singh MC, Raheja D. Help seeking behaviour of psychiatric patients before seeking care at a mental hospital. Int J Soc Psychiatry. 2001;47:71–8. https://doi.org/10.1177/002076400104700406.

Chakraborty K, Thakurata RG. Indian concepts on sexuality. Indian J Psychiatry. 2013;55:S250–5. https://doi.org/10.4103/0019-5545.105546.

De Silva P, Dissanayake SAW. The loss of Semen syndrome in Sri Lanka: a clinical study. Sex Marital Ther. 1989;4:195–204. https://doi.org/10.1080/02674658908408337.

Goldberg DP, Huxley P. Mental illness in the community: the pathway to psychiatric care. Psychology Press; 2001.

Grover S, Gupta S, Mehra A, Avasthi A. Comorbidity, knowledge and attitude towards sex among patients with Dhat syndrome: a retrospective study. Asian J Psychiatr. 2015;17:50–5. https://doi.org/10.1016/j.ajp.2015.07.002.

Grover S, Avasthi A, Gupta S, et al. Phenomenology and beliefs of patients with Dhat syndrome: a nationwide multicentric study. Int J Soc Psychiatry. 2016a;62:57–66. https://doi.org/10.1177/0020764015591857.

Grover S, Gupta S, Mahajan S, Avasthi A. Pathway of care among patients with Dhat syndrome attending a psychosexual clinic in tertiary care center in North India. Ind Psychiatry J. 2016b;25:72. https://doi.org/10.4103/0972-6748.196040.

Kar SK, Sarkar S. Dhat syndrome: evolution of concept, current understanding, and need of an integrated approach. J Hum Reprod Sci. 2015;8:130–4. https://doi.org/10.4103/0974-1208.165143.

Kar SK, Singh A. Person centered management approach for the Dhat syndrome. Int J Pers Cent Med. 2016;6. https://doi.org/10.5750/ijpcm.v6i4.615.

Kar GC, Varma LP. Sexual problems of married male mental patients. Indian J Psychiatry. 1978;20:365.

Kar S, Menon V, Arafat SM, et al. Dhat syndrome: systematic review of epidemiology, nosology, clinical features, and management strategies. Asian J Psychiatr. 2021;65:102863. https://doi.org/10.1016/j.ajp.2021.102863.

Kendurkar A, Kaur B, Agarwal AK, et al. Profile of adult patients attending a marriage and sex clinic in India. Int J Soc Psychiatry. 2008;54:486–93. https://doi.org/10.1177/0020764008090795.

Khan N. Dhat syndrome in relation to demographic characteristics. Indian J Psychiatry. 2005;47:54. https://doi.org/10.4103/0019-5545.46077.

Prakash O, Kar SK, Sathyanarayana Rao TS. Indian story on semen loss and related Dhat syndrome. Indian J Psychiatry. 2014;56:377. https://doi.org/10.4103/0019-5545.146532.

Prakash S, Sharan P, Sood M. A qualitative study on psychopathology of dhat syndrome in men: implications for classification of disorders. Asian J Psychiatr. 2018;35:79–88. https://doi.org/10.1016/j.ajp.2018.05.007.
Ranjith G, Mohan R. Dhat syndrome as a functional somatic syndrome: developing a sociosomatic model. Psychiatry. 2006;69:142–50. https://doi.org/10.1521/psyc.2006.69.2.142.
Rogler LH, Cortes DE. Help-seeking pathways: a unifying concept in mental health care. Am J Psychiatry. 1993;150:554–61. https://doi.org/10.1176/ajp.150.4.554.
Shahi MK, Tripathi A, Singh A, et al. Quality of life and disability in patients with dhat syndrome: a cross-sectional study. Indian J Psychol Med. 2022;44:459–65. https://doi.org/10.1177/02537176221078422.
Shoib S, Das S, Singhal S, et al. Dhat syndrome—a culture-bound sex neurosis of the Indian subcontinent: a prospective randomized study. Int J Cult Ment Health. 2018;11:470–7. https://doi.org/10.1080/17542863.2018.1427769.
Singh G. Dhat syndrome revisited. Indian J Psychiatry. 1985;27:119–22.
Singh A, Tripathi A, Gupta B, Agarwal V. Pathways to care for Dhat (Semen loss anxiety) syndrome: a study from North India. Int J Ment Health. 2016;45:253–61. https://doi.org/10.1080/00207411.2016.1238741.
Sorketti EA, Zuraida NZ, Habil MH. Pathways to mental healthcare in high-income and low-income countries. Int Psychiatry. 2013;10:45–7.
Verma RK, Sharma S, Singh R, et al. Beliefs concerning sexual health problems and treatment seeking among men in an Indian slum community. Cult Health Sex. 2003;5:265–76. https://doi.org/10.1080/136910501106356.

# Chapter 8
# Assessment of Dhat Syndrome: Clinical to Behavioral

**Sandeep Grover**

## 8.1 Introduction

Dhat syndrome is understood as a culture-bound syndrome that is characterized by preoccupation with the loss of semen. The condition was first described by Prof N. N. Wig, who observed that the patients with this syndrome are preoccupied with the excessive loss of semen. The perceived loss of semen is associated with guilt, which often leads to undue concern about the debilitating effect of semen loss on physical and psychological health. Persons with this syndrome commonly present with vague somatic symptoms such as fatigue, weakness, anxiety, loss of appetite, guilt, and sexual dysfunction that is attributed by the sufferer to loss of semen in nocturnal emission, in urine, or by masturbation (Wig 1960).

Over the years, many studies have been conducted to understand the symptom profile of patients with Dhat syndrome (Avasthi et al. 2012). It is now understood to be more common among young men. In recent times a female equivalent has also been described (Grover et al. 2014a, 2016a).

Vague and multiple somatic and psychological symptoms like lack of physical strength, fatigue, listlessness, poor concentration, forgetfulness, etc., characterize the usual clinical presentation of Dhat syndrome in males. The core feature is the undue concern with the passage of semen during micturition or while straining to pass stools, despite the lack of objective evidence of semen in urine or its passage otherwise (Avasthi et al. 2012). Dhat syndrome is commonly associated with comorbid psychiatric disorders and sexual dysfunctions (Grover et al. 2015a, b).

S. Grover (✉)
Department of Psychiatry, Post Graduate Institute of Medical Education and Research, Chandigarh, India

© The Author(s), under exclusive license to Springer Nature Singapore Pte Ltd. 2024

S. K. Kar et al. (eds.), *Dhat Syndrome*,
https://doi.org/10.1007/978-981-99-8870-9_8

In terms of nosology, Dhat Syndrome was listed under the category of "other specified nonpsychotic neurotic disorders" (F48.8) in the International Classification of Diseases (ICD-10) (World Health Organization (WHO) 1992) and the Diagnostic and Statistical Manual of Mental Disorders (DSM-IV-R) classified it as a "culture-bound syndrome." (American Psychiatric Association (APA) 2004). However, the DSM-5 considers Dhat syndrome a "cultural concept of distress" under the glossary section (American Psychiatric Association (APA, 2013).

A thorough assessment of a patient with Dhat syndrome is paramount in carrying out the required interventions. This chapter discusses the critical issues that must be considered while assessing a male patient presenting with Dhat syndrome. A brief note will also be made about the assessment of females presenting with the female equivalent of the Dhat syndrome.

For proper assessment, it is essential to understand the clinical picture of patients presenting with Dhat syndrome. Accordingly, the first section of the chapter discusses the clinical presentation of Dhat syndrome, and a detailed assessment follows this.

## 8.2 Clinical Features of Dhat Syndrome

Patients with Dhat syndrome usually present to clinicians with complaints of generalized weakness that they attribute to the loss of semen, either by night falls or loss of semen in urine. Occasional patients may also report loss of semen through the anus. These patients present with various symptoms ranging from affective, somatic, behavioural, depressive cognitions, neuro-cognitive and sexual symptoms (Fig. 8.1 and Table 8.1). Different studies vary in reporting these symptoms. Earlier studies have assessed the range of symptoms based on spontaneous reporting or self-designed scales. Recently, some studies have used various standard scales for assessing depression, anxiety, and somatic symptoms and have broadened the range of symptoms. In general, the affective symptoms include sadness, apprehension, worries (related to future sexual performance, being about father a child, becoming impotent, etc.), irritability, and anxiety. The somatic symptoms include generalized weakness, body aches, lethargy, low energy, tiredness, listlessness, burning micturition, turbid micturition, night falls, etc.

Regarding behavioural change, the patients usually report being withdrawn, having reduced sleep, reduced appetite, reduced libido, change in the masturbatory or sexual practices to conserve semen, etc. These patients also have significant depressive cognitions or cognitive errors in the form of preoccupation with semen loss, negative views about the future, catastrophization, preoccupation with change in their appearance, etc. Patients also complain of neurocognitive symptoms such as poor attention and concentration, forgetfulness, and their brain not functioning properly due to semen loss. The sexual symptoms may include a change in the masturbatory or sexual practices to conserve semen, masturbatory guilt, pain or problems during sexual intercourse, distress related to having night falls, premature

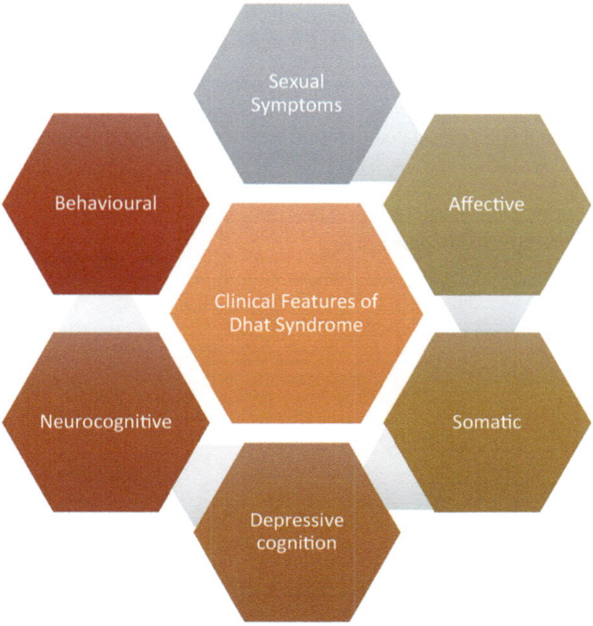


**Fig. 8.1** Clinical features of Dhat syndrome

ejaculation, erectile dysfunction, and perceived change in the size of the genitals (Table 8.1).

The most crucial aspect of Dhat syndrome is the attribution of all these symptoms to loss of semen. Additionally, these patients may have associated beliefs related to the formation of semen and the impact of the loss of semen on the body in general, sexual functioning, sexual potency, etc. A significant proportion of the patients with Dhat syndrome also have psychiatric comorbidity and sexual dysfunction (Table 8.2) (Grover et al. 2014a, b, 2016a, b; Kar et al. 2021; Prakash et al. 2016; Strong et al. 2022).

A syndrome similar to Dhat syndrome has also been reported in females that presents as nonpathological leukorrhea or vaginal discharge associated with the belief that they are losing vital fluid from the body. The clinical presentation includes affective, somatic, depressive cognition, neurocognitive symptoms, and behavioural symptoms similar to those seen in males. In terms of sexual symptoms, this may be associated with decreased libido. In contrast to males, the majority of these females also report the passage of vaginal discharge occurring spontaneously (i.e., not related to any specific situation); however, some of them report the occurrence of vaginal discharge while straining for stools, while passing urine, during sexual excitement, while watching/reading pornography, and just before or after menstruation and while experiencing sexual dreams (Grover et al. 2016a, b, 2014a, b; Mehra et al. 2021; Joshi et al. 2022).

**Table 8.1** Common symptoms observed in patients with Dhat syndrome (Grover et al. 2014a, b, 2016a, b; Kar et al. 2021; Prakash et al. 2016; Strong et al. 2022)

| |
|---|
| **Affective symptoms** |
| • Sadness of mood |
| • Apprehension and worries (related to future sexual performance, fathering a child, becoming impotent, etc.) |
| • Irritability |
| • Anxiety (generalized or related to sexual performance in the future) |
| • Little interest or pleasure in doing things |
| **Somatic symptoms** |
| • Generalized body weakness |
| • Body aches |
| • Stomach ache |
| • Back pain |
| • Pain in arms, legs, or joints |
| • Feeling tired or having low energy |
| • Lethargy |
| • Listlessness |
| • Burning micturition |
| • Turbid micturition |
| • Headaches |
| • Chest pain |
| • Dizziness |
| • Fainting spells |
| • Feeling heart pound or race |
| • Shortness of breath |
| • Constipation, loose bowels, or diarrhoea |
| • Nausea, gas, or indigestion |
| • Restlessness/psychomotor retardation |
| **Thoughts** |
| • Preoccupation with semen loss |
| • Negative view about future |
| • Other depressive cognitions |
| • Catastrophization |
| • Preoccupation with change in their appearance |
| **Behavioural symptoms** |
| • Social withdrawal |
| • Disturbed sleep |
| • Reduced appetite |
| • Lack of libido or having normal libido |
| **Cognitive symptoms** |
| • Forgetfulness |
| • Poor attention and concentration |
| • Mental weakness/fatigue |
| **Sexual symptoms** |
| • Change in the masturbatory or sexual practices to conserve semen |
| • Masturbatory guilt |
| • Pain or problems during sexual intercourse |
| • Night falls |
| • Premature ejaculation |
| • Erectile dysfunction |
| • Perceived change in the size of the genitals |

## 8.3 Assessment of Patients Presenting with Dhat Syndrome

Proper management of patients presenting with Dhat syndrome requires detailed assessment. The detailed assessment can also guide the clinicians about the areas to focus on while psychoeducation. Accordingly, assessment should not focus on clinical features only but also should focus on understanding the patient's beliefs about the loss of semen, sources of such beliefs, how much the patient believes in such information and myths associated with the semen loss (Avasthi et al. 2017).

A detailed scheme of assessment of persons presenting with Dhat syndrome is presented in Table 8.2. While taking history, the clinicians should make a note of the age of onset of symptoms, the whole range of symptoms, attribution of symptoms (i.e., loss of semen to be responsible for the various symptoms), frequency of semen loss, consistency and quantity of semen loss, situations in which semen loss occurs, beliefs and myths related to why they have semen loss, understanding about the semen formation, sources of (mis)information about semen formation, perceived consequences of loss of Dhat, sexual practices since the beginning and any change in sexual practices since the onset of clinical features. Additionally, the clinicians should also focus on any sexual encounters and patients' performance during the sexual encounter, night falls, any sexual dysfunction, comorbid psychiatric disorders, and comorbid physical diseases. An important aspect of assessment also includes obtaining a treatment history, including the pathways of care followed by the patient to date, as often many of the myths of patients are either reinforced or are attributed to the traditional healers. Further, assessing the patient's expectations from the treatment is essential, i.e., whether they think medications will help them or some counselling would be helpful. This is important because if the clinicians try to manage these patients without understanding their expectations from the treatment, then it is very likely that these patients will drop out of the treatment (Grover et al. 2014a, b, 2016a, b; Kar et al. 2021; Prakash et al. 2016; Strong et al. 2022).

The scheme of assessment for female Dhat syndrome is also similar. However, while evaluating such females, it is essential to rule out any vaginal infection, and it is always better to investigate. In terms of consequences of vaginal discharge, females with Dhat syndrome may report weakness in the body, reduced stamina, body thinness, poor sexual ability, experiencing repeated vaginal infection, mental illness, pain in genital areas, loss of beauty of face and body, menstrual problems, and irritability before or after menstruation (Grover et al. 2016a, 2014a; Mehra et al. 2021; Joshi et al. 2022).

The assessment of Dhat syndrome can be done through history taking, mental status examination, and physical examination. However, specific questionnaires and interviews have recently been developed to collect information about various aspects of Dhat syndrome in both males and females (Grover et al. 2014b, 2016a; Prakash et al. 2016). The clinician can also use screening questionnaires for depression, anxiety and somatic symptoms to broaden the assessment. In the subsequent section, we discuss the questionnaires/interviews specifically designed to assess Dhat Syndrome.

**Table 8.2** Assessment for patients with Dhat syndrome

| | |
|---|---|
| History taking | • **Age of onset of symptoms**<br>• **Symptoms:** Affective, Somatic, Behavioural, Depressive cognitions, Neurocognition, Sexual<br>• **Attribution of symptoms**<br>• **Frequency of semen loss**<br>• **Consistency and quantity of semen loss**<br>• **Beliefs & Myths related to semen loss (reasons for passage of Dhat):** Excessive masturbation, excessive sexual intercourse, due to sexual intercourse with a woman while she was menstruating, premarital sexual intercourse, due to sexual intercourse outside wedlock, homosexual relationship, sexual intercourse with commercial sex workers, sexual intercourse in an unnatural way, sexual dreams, low/excessive sexual desire, lack of indulgence in masturbation, eating unbalanced food/absurd food, excessive eating, wrong deeds of past life, lack of sleep/improper sleep, constipation, worm infestation of the gastrointestinal tract, urinary infection or problems of the urinary tract, hereditary reasons (because others in family also suffer from the same problem)<br>• **Knowledge about how semen formation occurs**<br>• **Source(s) of information about semen formation**<br>• **Situations in which they experience loss of Dhat:** Micturition, defecation, night falls/nocturnal emissions, passive stimulation, sexual intercourse<br>• **Sexual practices (masturbation/sexual intercourse), including change in the sexual practices with the emergence of features of Dhat syndrome**<br>• **Sexual encounters and performance**<br>• **History of night falls and reasons for the same**<br>• **Perceived consequences of loss of Dhat:** Weakness in sexual ability, negative impact on physical appearance, malformation of children, more chances of having a female child, early death<br>• **Comorbid sexual dysfunction:** Premature ejaculation, erectile dysfunction, change in the size of the genitals<br>• **Comorbid psychiatric disorders:** Depression, dysthymia, mixed anxiety and depressive disorder, adjustment disorder, somatoform disorder, Generalized anxiety disorder, obsessive-compulsive disorder, and other anxiety disorders<br>• **Comorbid physical diseases**<br>• **Treatment history, including pathways of care**<br>• **Expectations from treatment** |
| Physical examination | • General physical examination to rule out any possible physical illness<br>• Genital examination for any infection, size of genitals |
| Mental status examination | • Evaluate for depressive disorders, anxiety disorders, somatic symptoms |
| Investigations | • Urine examination: Routine & Microscopy<br>• Other investigations: Guided by the history and physical examination |

### 8.3.1 Comprehensive Questionnaire for Assessment of Dhat Syndrome

This questionnaire was developed by Grover et al. (2014a, b). The original scale was designed in Hindi and was then translated into English. The questionnaire has multiple choice questions with 'yes/no' responses and specific responses in various other rating formats, and open-ended questions covering various symptoms (duration of passage of Dhat, frequency of passage of Dhat, the quantity of semen (Dhat) lost each time, colour and consistency of the Dhat, and associated somatic symptoms), beliefs/myths related to Dhat (content and composition, situation/time of passage of Dhat, perceived causes of passage of Dhat, and perceived consequences of Dhat) and beliefs and behaviour related to treatment (Grover et al. 2014a, b). This questionnaire has been reported to have adequate face validity. The Hindi and English versions have been shown to have good cross-language equivalence. The Hindi version has been shown to have good test -retest validity when completed by the same subjects on two separate occasions after a few days. This scale has been translated into many other Indian languages, such as Punjabi, Kannada, Bengali, Oriya, Gujarati, Marathi, Tamil, and Telugu, by using the World Health Organization methodology of translation and back translation (Grover et al, 2016b). This questionnaire has been used in many recent studies and the only multicentric study on Dhat syndrome conducted in India (Grover et al, 2016b). The female equivalent of this questionnaire is known as Scale for Assessment of Female Dhat Syndrome (SAFED) (Grover et al. 2016a).

### 8.3.2 Dhat Disorder Diagnostic Interview

This diagnostic interview consists of seven questions designed to assess the diagnostic criteria of the syndrome, with the assessment period being last several weeks (Prakash et al. 2016).

### 8.3.3 Dhat Syndrome Severity Scale

This questionnaire has different sections. The initial section includes a description of the belief and its cause over the last week, followed by questions to rule out alternative causes and the mode of the passage of Dhat. This is followed by a section on health beliefs that lists 25 health belief dimensions derived from scales used to describe firmly held beliefs such as overvalued ideas, delusions, and culture-bound syndromes. Each item is rated from zero to three. The final section of the scale includes a list of 139 symptoms and items to rate the overall distress and dysfunction on a scale of zero to three as per the clinician's judgment (Prakash et al. 2016).

## 8.4 Conclusion

To conclude, assessment of Dhat syndrome requires a detailed review of history in terms of symptoms, myths and beliefs, help-seeking, consequences and reviewing the psychiatric symptoms. Additionally, the clinicians should also carry out a detailed physical examination and mental status examination for ruling out other causes and for evaluating comorbidities. Questionnaires specific to the assessment of Dhat syndrome should be used to have a comprehensive understanding of the patients and this can also guide the management of Dhat Syndrome.

## References

American Psychiatric Association (APA). Diagnostic and statistical manual of mental disorders. 4th ed, text rev. Washington: American Psychiatric Publishing; 2004.

American Psychiatric Association (APA). Diagnostic and statistical manual of mental disorders. 5th ed. Washington: American Psychiatric Publishing; 2013.

Avasthi A, Grover S, Jhirwal OP. Dhat syndrome: a culture-bound sex related disorder in Indian subcontinent. In: Gupta S, Kumar B, editors. Sexually transmitted infections. 2nd ed. New Delhi, India: Elsevier; 2012. p. 1225–30.

Avasthi A, Grover S, Sathyanarayana Rao TS. Clinical practice guidelines for management of sexual dysfunction. Indian J Psychiatry. 2017;59(Suppl 1):S91–S115.

Grover S, Avasthi A, Aneja J, Shankar G, Mohan MR, Nehra R, Padhy SK. Comprehensive questionnaire for the assessment of Dhat syndrome: development and use in the patient population. J Sex Med. 2014b;11(10):2485–95.

Grover S, Avasthi A, Gupta S, Dan A, Neogi R, Behere PB, Lakdawala B, Tripathi A, Chakraborty K, Sinha V, Bhatia MS, Patjoshi A, Rao TS, Rozatkar A. Phenomenology and beliefs of patients with Dhat syndrome: a nationwide multicentric study. Int J Soc Psychiatry. 2016b;62(1):57–66.

Grover S, Avasthi A, Gupta S, Dan A, Neogi R, Behere PB, Lakdawala B, Tripathi A, Chakraborty K, Sinha V, Bhatia MS, Pattojoshi A, Rao TS, Rozatkar A. Comorbidity in patients with Dhat syndrome: a nationwide multicentric study. J Sex Med. 2015b;12(6):1398–401.

Grover S, Avasthi A, Gupta S, Hazari N, Malhotra N. Do female patients with nonpathological vaginal discharge need the same evaluation as for Dhat syndrome in males? Indian J Psychiatry. 2016a;58:61–9.

Grover S, Gupta S, Mehra A, Avasthi A. Comorbidity, knowledge and attitude towards sex among patients with Dhat syndrome: a retrospective study. Asian J Psychiatr. 2015a;17:50–5.

Grover S, Kate N, Avasthi A, Rajpal N, Umamaheswari V. Females too suffer from Dhat syndrome: a case series and revisit of the concept. Indian J Psychiatry. 2014a;56(4):388–92.

Joshi S, Tripathi A, Agarwal S, Singh N, Gupta B, Nischal A, Kar SK. Phenomenology, disability and sexual functioning in female Dhat syndrome: a study of tertiary care gynecology outpatients. Gen Psychiatr. 2022;35(5):e100863.

Kar SK, Menon V, Arafat SY, Singh A, Das A, Shankar A, Sharma P, Perera S. Dhat syndrome: systematic review of epidemiology, nosology, clinical features, and management strategies. Asian J Psychiatr. 2021;65:102863.

Mehra A, Kathirvel S, Gainder S, Avasthi A, Grover S. Female Dhat syndrome in primary care setting. Ind Psychiatry J. 2021;30(2):278–84.

Prakash S, Sharan P, Sood M. A study on phenomenology of Dhat syndrome in men in a general medical setting. Indian J Psychiatry. 2016;58:129–41.

Strong YN, Li A, White ME, Razzak AN, Anderson DJ, Kaye AD, Herron EW, Khater NP, Bradley EC, Urits I. Dhat syndrome: epidemiology, risk factors, comorbidities, diagnosis, treatment, and management. Health Psychol Res. 2022;10(4):38759.
Wig N. Problems of mental health in India. J Clin Soc Psychiatry. 1960;17:48–53.
World Health Organization (WHO). The ICD-10 classification of mental and behavioral disorders: diagnostic criteria for research. Geneva: WHO; 1992.

# Chapter 9
# Entities that Mimic Dhat Syndrome

**Yukino N. Strong**

## 9.1 Dhat Syndrome Worldwide

Dhat syndrome is currently classified as a culture-bound syndrome in both the ICD-10 and DSM-5, due to its prevalence in India and connection to ancient Ayurvedic texts (Kar and Sarkar 2015). However, we find that similar syndromes with different names exist in many other Asian cultures. Some examples include "prameha" in Sri Lanka, "shen k'uei" in China, "latah" in Malayo-Indonesia, and "imu" in Japan (Deb and Balhara 2013). While Dhat syndrome is thought to be a primarily Eastern syndrome, there are historical records of similar syndromes in the Western world. Both Galen and Aristotle make mention of the detrimental effects of excessive semen loss. Many western religions including Christianity, Catholicism, and Judaism prohibit masturbation and premarital sex just as Hinduism and other Vedic religions do, creating opportunity for guilt related to both of those activities (Deb and Balhara 2013). Prominent early American psychiatrists Benjamin Rush and Sylvester Graham noted a syndrome of physical fatigue they attributed to excessive loss of semen (Sumithipala et al. 2004). A study conducted by Shahi et al. (2022) found that patients with Dhat syndrome have statistically significant lower quality of life than healthy patients, including patients without other comorbidities. They also found that the relationship between quality of life and distress was bidirectional: leaving Dhat syndrome untreated decreased quality of life further and that decreased quality of life correlated with an increase in distress over semen loss (Shahi et al. 2022).

In 2013, a study conducted in a Spanish urology speciality clinic found that of 396 new patients, 32 of them had a primary complaint of semen loss (Menéndez et al. 2013). Thirty of these men were from Pakistan, with two from Bangladesh. Although Spain is not traditionally a country where Dhat syndrome is prevalent, it

Y. N. Strong (✉)
Central Medical Maine Center Family Medicine, Lewiston, ME, USA

© The Author(s), under exclusive license to Springer Nature Singapore Pte Ltd. 2024
S. K. Kar et al. (eds.), *Dhat Syndrome*,
https://doi.org/10.1007/978-981-99-8870-9_9

is expected that as travel becomes more common and the world more homogenized, even physicians in the West will see patients with Dhat syndrome. Combined with the historical precedent set by many prominent physicians spanning America, England, France, and Australia in the nineteenth century who held strong beliefs regarding the effects of excessive semen lost through activities other than marital sex and treated patients accordingly (Sumithipala et al. 2004), it would be unwise to dismiss Dhat syndrome as a purely eastern syndrome. Physicians worldwide should be educated on the diagnosis and management of Dhat syndrome as it becomes increasingly likely that they will encounter these patients in clinical settings. In order to correctly diagnose and treat these patients, it is important to rule out other entities that mimic Dhat syndrome.

## 9.2 Entities that Mimic Dhat Syndrome

### *9.2.1 Infections*

One 26-year-old male presented with the prototypical symptoms of Dhat syndrome. He complained of a "spoonful" of penile discharge that was milky-colored and occurring multiple times a day with and without triggers. This coincided with a stressful life experience, and he reported many psychiatric symptoms. Along with these, he complained of many vague somatic symptoms such as body aches, nausea, and dizziness. After seeking treatment from multiple traditional faith healers, he sought help from a private clinic. They diagnosed his symptoms as a urinary tract infection and prescribed him antibiotics (MacFarland et al. 2017).

As with all psychiatric syndromes, organic causes must be ruled out when diagnosing Dhat syndrome. Infections are one culprit whose symptoms overlap with Dhat syndrome. Gautham et al. (2008) collected urine samples from 366 men presenting to local provider clinics in India with complaints of dhat, burning or painful micturition, involuntary nocturnal emissions, turbid urine, genital itching, and genital ulcers or boils. Of these symptomatic men, about 5.5% of them were found positive for either chlamydia trachomatis or Neisseria gonorrhoea.

Other studies postulating that the symptoms of dhat can be attributed to either sexually transmitted or urinary tract infections have examined urine and found phosphaturia, oxaluria, pus cells, and alkaline urine (Deb and Balhara 2013). Any one of these may contribute to the turbid urine that distresses patients so much.

### 9.2.2 *Postorgasmic Illness Syndrome*

Postorgasmic illness syndrome (POIS) is a poorly understood syndrome in which patients present with a range of flu-like symptoms post-ejaculation (Ashby and Goldmeier 2010). These symptoms usually present within 30 minutes of ejaculation, peak around 12–48 hours after, and can last up to 7 days (Rosetti et al. 2023). One theory of the mechanism of POIS is an autoimmune or allergic response. Another is that it is an inflammatory response (Rosetti et al. 2023).

Ashby and Goldmeier (2010) compare two patients; one diagnosed with POIS and the other with Dhat syndrome. The first patient was a 57-year-old male who had sex with men, had been with his partner for 10 years, and had been experiencing symptoms for 6 years. He reported symptoms of both physical and mental fatigue, myalgias in his legs, right-sided headache, excessive sweating, and poor concentration. The symptoms reached a point where the patient began avoiding sex out of fear of experiencing these symptoms. The researchers performed multiple tests including bloodwork, an electrocardiogram (ECG), autonomic testing, and a Magnetic Resonance Image (MRI) of the brain, all of which had normal results. They also administered repeated neuropsychological testing and a Hospital Anxiety and Depression Score (HADS). The neuropsychological testing on day 1 and day 2 after orgasm did not show any significant difference compared to his baseline. He also scored low on HADS, so it was concluded he did not have comorbid depression or anxiety. As no other cause was found for his symptoms, researchers prescribed him 75 mg of diclofenac to take 1–2 h before orgasm and for 1–2 days after, as the proposed mechanisms of POIS include an inflammatory reaction. The patient reported an 80% improvement in his symptoms with the medication (Ashby and Goldmeier 2010).

The second patient was a 27-year-old Pakistani male who had a prior history of sex with men but who identified as heterosexual at the time of the study. He had a female partner for 1 year when he presented to the clinic. His symptoms were not consistent every time he experienced orgasm; they were reported to be less severe when he was able to maintain an erection long enough to achieve vaginal penetration. This patient underwent the same testing as the first, again with no abnormal results. His HADS was negative. However, his neuropsychological testing did show some decline in simple reaction time, perceptual motor speed, and psychomotor speed 1 h after orgasm compared to 5 days after orgasm. The researchers trialed diclofenac on this patient as well; however, he experienced no relief from his symptoms. They then began treatment for his erectile dysfunction and his postorgasmic symptoms resolved as well. This lead them to believe the symptoms were due to Dhat syndrome rather than POIS (Ashby and Goldmeier 2010).

Patients with these two syndromes present with remarkably similar symptoms of weakness and other somatic symptoms following orgasm. If the physician is unable to distinguish which one the patient is experiencing, it seems reasonable to trial a potent nonsteroidal anti-inflammatory drug and monitor for resolution of symptoms. This would rule out Dhat syndrome and confirm POIS.

### 9.2.3 *Pelvic Disorders*

It is now known that females too may suffer from Dhat syndrome. Much less is known about the presentation of female Dhat syndrome and literature on the topic is lacking. Mehra et al. (2021) surveyed 69 women at an outpatient gynecology clinic in a rural area. All of the women were found to have nonpathological vaginal discharge and were evaluated using the Scale for Assessment of Female Dhat syndrome (SAFeD). The patients attributed many of the same somatic symptoms as males typically do to the loss of dhat. Some uniquely reported pain in the genitals, both during and not related to sexual activity (Mehra et al. 2021). This brings to mind some pelvic disorders that may be mistakenly labelled as Dhat syndrome, especially in females.

Vaginismus and dyspareunia both typically present as pain during the vaginal examination. Unlike Dhat syndrome, they also characteristically have elevated vaginal and/or pelvic muscle tone (Lahaie et al. 2010). Dyspareunia and vaginismus can often be differentiated from each other by the characteristics of the pain they are experiencing. With vaginismus, there is thought to be a component of fear or anxiety, leading to significantly increased efforts to avoid penetrative activities compared to women with dyspareunia (Lahaie et al. 2010). This experience of genital pain with psychological features is similar to the presentation of Dhat syndrome in women; thus physicians need to be able to determine what specifically is causing their patients distress in the situation.

Chronic pelvic pain syndrome is another syndrome with a poorly understood etiology. It is simply characterized by pain localized to the pelvis for longer than 6 months, whether cyclic or noncyclic (Polackwich and Shoskes 2016). Many potential factors contribute, including psychosomatic. The treatment for chronic pelvic pain syndrome ranges from analgesics to hormones to surgery (Polackwich and Shoskes 2016). Again, physicians must assess for Dhat syndrome which can be treated through education before performing life-altering surgery to cure what they believe to be chronic pelvic pain syndrome.

### 9.2.4 *Koro Syndrome*

Koro syndrome is a culture-bound syndrome similar to Dhat syndrome. It is defined by a belief that one's external genitalia are shrinking. In fact, Koro is believed to be derived from the Malay word for "head of a turtle" (Mattelaer and Jilek 2007) Accompanying this fear is the belief that shrunken genitalia can lead to sexual dysfunction, infertility, and ultimately death. Koro syndrome is most prevalent in China but has been seen across Asia, Africa, and medieval Europe (Mattelaer and Jilek 2007). The cause of Koro syndrome is usually attributed to folklore specific to the geographical area, including but not limited to female fox spirits, sorcerers, and witches (Mattelaer and Jilek 2007).

Like Dhat syndrome, there is a lack of literature on Koro syndrome. The consensus on the treatment appears to be a combination of psychotherapy with a sexual education component paired with antidepressants or anxiolytics (Strong et al. 2023). As the treatment is the same for Koro syndrome as it is for Dhat syndrome, the area of focus for the physician should be on the underlying cause of the anxiety to anticipate possible compensatory behaviours their patients may engage in. With Koro syndrome, there have been cases of patients attaching apparatuses to their genitalia to prevent shrinkage (Strong et al. 2023), whereas there have been documented cases of patients with Dhat syndrome drinking their semen to prevent semen loss (Agrawal et al. 2022). As the physician is aware of the detailed differences between Dhat syndrome and Koro syndrome they can proactively counsel patients against unhelpful behaviors.

## 9.3 Three Categories of Dhat Syndrome

Studies often characterize Dhat syndrome into three categories: Dhat syndrome with comorbid psychiatric diagnoses, Dhat syndrome with comorbid sexual dysfunction, and Dhat syndrome alone (Grover et al. 2015a, b). This is important to be aware of as patients may present with either psychiatric symptoms or sexual dysfunction and not be fully treated with traditional therapies until the dhat component is addressed as well.

### *9.3.1 Dhat Syndrome with Comorbid Psychiatric Diagnoses*

Experts have not come to a consensus on the issue of Dhat syndrome being a cultural manifestation of depression or anxiety, a somatoform disorder, or a completely separate diagnosis (Dhikav et al. 2008). One study with 30 patients with Dhat syndrome found that 20 of them had varying symptoms of depression, as measured by the Hamilton depression scale (Dhikav et al. 2008). Another study looked at 106 patients with Dhat syndrome and no previously diagnosed psychiatric comorbidities (Grover et al. 2015a, b). They found that 13.2% filled the criteria for a depressive disorder, while 15.1% filled the criteria for any of the anxiety disorders. They then compared the group with Dhat syndrome with no comorbidities with healthy patient controls from the same clinic. When comparing these two groups, there was no statistically significant difference in the hypochondriasis scale. However, the depression alone group was found to score significantly higher on two out of three alexithymia scales.

Grover et al. (2015a, b) then compared the Dhat syndrome alone group with a group of patients from the same clinic who had a somatoform disorder only. They found that the Dhat syndrome alone group scored significantly higher on somatosensory amplification. The somatoform-only group scored higher on the hypochondriasis scale.

Patients were sorted into mild, moderate, and severe Dhat syndrome categories based on the presentation of their symptoms. They found no correlation between the severity of Dhat syndrome and the presence of a comorbid psychiatric disorder (Grover et al. 2015a, b).

However, Dhat syndrome can either manifest or be mistaken for other psychiatric disorders. One 19-year-old female began experiencing low energy and body aches shortly after developing nonpathological vaginal discharge (Grover et al. 2014). Six months later, thoughts of dhat being "dirty" became intrusive and unstoppable. She would repeatedly ask other females if they too were experiencing symptoms. She also began compulsively washing her genitalia. She eventually sought psychiatric care and was diagnosed with both Dhat syndrome and obsessive-compulsive disorder. With medication and psychoeducation to target both aspects of her psychiatric disorders, her symptomology of both improved by approximately 80%.

Similar to the way a schizophrenic prodrome can present as a depressive episode, one Hindu male experienced Dhat syndrome as a prodrome to schizophrenia (Kar et al. 2017). He began to complain about the loss of dhat at age 15. He attributed his loss of energy, anxiety, weight loss, poor concentration, etc. to his loss of semen. Six months later, he began having delusions of persecution and reference. He married at age 20 and experienced premature ejaculation with his wife, which he also attributed to the loss of dhat in early life. At 23, he went missing for a month and was found to have neck lacerations, at which point he was hospitalized and diagnosed with schizophrenia.

Rajkumar and Bharadwaj (2014) postulated that depression may sometimes be incorrectly characterized as Dhat syndrome. They studied 46 males with Dhat syndrome and split them into two groups: one with a positive family history of Dhat syndrome and one with a negative family history of Dhat syndrome. All of the demographic information that was collected for the study was the same across both groups, except for those with positive family histories who had fewer years of education on average. The positive family history group had statistically significant higher rates of both depressive disorders and substance use disorders. They argue that this correlation between positive family history and higher rates of depressive and/or substance use disorders may be evidence that Dhat syndrome is heritable; therefore, it is merely a subtype of depression and not its own diagnosis.

Contrary to this, we find three case studies where patients were diagnosed with either schizophrenia or major depressive disorder (Aneja et al. 2015). In all three cases, patients received pharmacologic therapy targeted at their specific disorders for years and struggled with medication compliance. However, once they were educated about Dhat syndrome and normal reproductive anatomy and physiology, they each reported decreased anxiety over semen loss and improved their medication compliance. This is perhaps suggestive of Dhat syndrome being masked or overshadowed by more defined psychiatric conditions. The physician needs to treat all aspects of a patient's condition. To do so, they must first be aware of all of the contributing factors.

### 9.3.2 Dhat Syndrome with Comorbid Sexual Dysfunction

Dhat syndrome is also commonly associated with sexual dysfunction. Studies have found up to 62% of patients with Dhat syndrome have erectile dysfunction and up to 44% experience premature ejaculation (Prakash and Rao 2010). When the pathways of care for patients with Dhat syndrome was examined, it was found that participants had an average of 2.85 other clinic visits before reaching the outpatient psychosexual clinic (Grover et al. 2016). They showed preference for visiting traditional faith healers, as well as general physicians, urologists, and surgeons. It is important for western practitioners of medicine to recognize the possibility of Dhat syndrome in a patient presenting to them for sexual dysfunction, as most patients will not present to a psychosexual clinic first.

### 9.3.3 "Pure" Dhat Syndrome

The third category is Dhat syndrome alone. It is still debated to this day if there is a "pure" version of Dhat syndrome. In a study comparing 32 Dhat syndrome patients with 33 healthy controls, the Somatization Screening Index (SSI), the screening version of the Illness Behavior Questionnaire (SIBQ), the Somatosensory Amplification Scale (SAS), the Whitley Index (WI), and the revised Chalder Fatigue Scale were administered (Perme et al. 2005). Of these, patients with Dhat syndrome scored significantly higher on the SSI, WI, and SIBQ, signifying higher levels of hypochondriacal beliefs, abnormal illness behaviour, somatic symptoms, and fatigue. These align with functional somatic syndromes as well, creating the argument that Dhat syndrome is merely a type of functional somatic syndrome.

A follow-up study on 41 patients with "pure" Dhat syndrome (no comorbidities) found that two thirds of them no longer fulfilled the criteria for Dhat syndrome. A quarter of them were in complete remission (Sameer et al. 2015). This lack of stability in diagnosis begs the question whether Dhat syndrome is a valid discrete diagnosis.

## 9.4 Conclusion

Whether or not Dhat syndrome is a stand-alone diagnosis, physicians everywhere must be informed about the signs and symptoms of this condition so they can deliver culturally-informed care to all of their patients. When presented with infections, postorgasmic illness syndrome, pelvic disorders, psychiatric symptoms, and sexual dysfunction, please consider Dhat syndrome in your differential diagnoses.

## References


Agrawal AK, Bagewadi V, Das S, Moirangthem S. Recycling of semen: a rare phenomenon in DHAT syndrome. Psychiatr Danub. 2022;34(2):313–4. https://doi.org/10.24869/psyd.2022.313.

Aneja J, Grover S, Avasthi A, Mahajan S, Pokhrel P, Triveni D. Can masturbatory guilt lead to severe psychopathology: a case series. Indian J Psychol Med. 2015;37(1):81–6. https://doi.org/10.4103/0253-7176.150848.

Ashby J, Goldmeier D. Postorgasm illness syndrome—a spectrum of illnesses. J Sex Med. 2010;7(5):1976–81. https://doi.org/10.1111/j.1743-6109.2010.01707.x.

Deb KS, Balhara YPS. Dhat syndrome: a review of the world literature. Indian J Psychol Med. 2013;35(4):326–31. https://doi.org/10.4103/0253-7176.122219.

Dhikav V, Aggarwal N, Gupta S, Jadhavi R, Singh K. Depression in Dhat syndrome. J Sex Med. 2008;5(4):841–4. https://doi.org/10.1111/j.1743-6109.2007.00481.x.

Gautham M, Singh R, Weiss H, Brugha R, Patel V, Desai NG, Nandan D, Kielmann K, Grosskurth H. Socio-cultural, psychosexual and biomedical factors associated with genital symptoms experienced by men in rural India. Tropical Med Int Health. 2008;13(3):384–95. https://doi.org/10.1111/J.1365-3156.2008.02013.X.

Grover S, Gupta S, Avasthi A. Psychological correlates and psychiatric morbidity in patients with Dhat syndrome. Indian J Psychiatry. 2015a;57(3):255–61. https://doi.org/10.4103/0019-5545.166637.

Grover S, Gupta S, Mahajan S, Avasthi A. Pathway of care among patients with Dhat syndrome attending a psychosexual clinic in tertiary care center in North India. Ind Psychiatry J. 2016;25(1):72–7. https://doi.org/10.4103/0972-6748.196040.

Grover S, Gupta S, Mehra A, Avasthi A. Comorbidity, knowledge and attitude towards sex among patients with Dhat syndrome: a retrospective study. Asian J Psychiatr. 2015b;17:50–5. https://doi.org/10.1016/j.ajp.2015.07.002.

Grover S, Kate N, Avasthi A, Rajpal N, Umamaheswari V. Females too suffer from Dhat syndrome: a case series and revisit of the concept. Indian J Psychiatry. 2014;56(4):388–92. https://doi.org/10.4103/0019-5545.146537.

Kar SK, Sarkar S. Dhat syndrome: evolution of concept, current understanding, and an integrated approach. J Hum Reprod Sci. 2015;8(3):130–4. https://doi.org/10.4103/0974-1208.165143.

Kar SK, Shahi MK, Tripathi A. Dhat syndrome as the prodrome of schizophrenia: understanding the cultural distress. Asian J Psychiatr. 2017;25:203–4. https://doi.org/10.1016/j.ajp.2016.11.006.

Lahaie MA, Boyer SC, Amsel R, Khalifé S, Binik YM. Vaginismus: a review of the literature on the classification/diagnosis, etiology and treatment. Women's Health (Lond Engl). 2010;6(5):705–19. https://doi.org/10.2217/WHE.10.46.

MacFarland AS, Al-Maashani M, Al Busaidi Q, Al-Naamani A, El-Bouri M, Al-Adawi S. Culture-specific pathogenicity of dhat (semen loss) syndrome in an Arab/Islamic society, Oman. Oman Med J. 2017;32(3):251–5. https://doi.org/10.5001/OMJ/2017.47.

Mattelaer JJ, Jilek W. Koro—the psychological disappearance of the penis. J Sex Med. 2007;4(5):1509–15. https://doi.org/10.1111/J.1743-6109.2007.00586.X.

Mehra A, Kathirvel S, Gainder S, Avasthi A, Grover S. Female Dhat syndrome in primary care setting. Ind Psychiatry J. 2021;30(2):278–84. https://doi.org/10.4103/ipj.ipj_76_20.

Menéndez V, Fernández-Suárez A, Placer J, García-Linares M, Tarragon S, Liso E. Dhat syndrome, an emergent condition within urology in Spain. World J Urol. 2013;31(4):941–5. https://doi.org/10.1007/S00345-012-0911-4.

Perme B, Ranjith G, Mohan R, Chandrasekaran R. Dhat (semen loss) syndrome: a functional somatic syndrome of the Indian subcontinent? Gen Hosp Psychiatry. 2005;27(3):215–7. https://doi.org/10.1016/j.genhosppsych.2005.01.003.

Polackwich AS, Shoskes DA. Chronic prostatitis/chronic pelvic pain syndrome: a review of evaluation and therapy. Prostate Cancer Prostatic Dis. 2016;19(2):132–8. https://doi.org/10.1038/PCAN.2016.8.

Prakash O, Rao TSS. Sexuality research in India: an update. Indian J Psychiatry. 2010;52(Suppl 1):S260–3. https://doi.org/10.4103/0019-5545.69243.

Rajkumar RP, Bharadwaj B. Dhat syndrome: evidence for a depressive spectrum subtype. Asian J Psychiatr. 2014;9:57–60. https://doi.org/10.1016/j.ajp.2014.01.007.

Rosetti L, Kanani A, Witherspoon L, Flannigan R, Elliott S. Case series: expanding diagnostic markers in postorgasmic illness syndrome. Sex Med. 2023;11(2):1–4. https://doi.org/10.1093/SEXMED/QFAC021.

Sameer M, Menon V, Chandrasekaran R. Is "pure" Dhat syndrome a stable diagnostic entity? A naturalistic long term follow up study from a tertiary care Centre. J Clin Diagn Res. 2015;9(8):VC01–3. https://doi.org/10.7860/JCDR/2015/13399.6275.

Shahi MK, Tripathi A, Singh A, Kar SK, Nischal A, Singh S, Dalal PK. Quality of life and disability in patients with Dhat syndrome: a cross-sectional study. Indian J Psychol Med. 2022;44(5):459–65. https://doi.org/10.1177/02537176221078422.

Strong YN, Cao DY, Zhou J, Guenther MA, Anderson DJ, Kaye AD, Blick BE, Anandi PR, Patel HY, Urits I. Koro syndrome: epidemiology, psychiatric and physical risk factors, clinical presentation, diagnosis, and treatment options. Health Psychol Res. 2023;11:70165. https://doi.org/10.5296/001c.70165.

Sumithipala A, Siribaddana SH, Bhugra D. Culture-bound syndromes: the story of dhat syndrome. Br J Psychiatry. 2004;184(MAR):200–9. https://doi.org/10.1192/bjp.184.3.200.

# Chapter 10
# Pharmacological Management of Dhat Syndrome

M. S. Bhatia and Aparna Goyal

## 10.1 Introduction

The word "Dhat" basically has its origin in Sanskrit language. In Sanskrit it is "dhatu" meaning a very important bodily substance needed for preservation of health and longevity. It is primarily a culture-bound syndrome more limited to South East Asian countries with some sporadic off shoots in different parts of the world. But again, it can be reported as those who immigrated from South East Asian regions (Strong et al. 2022).

Dhat syndrome is characterized by a spectrum of anxio-depressive-somato-cognitive manifestations that are attributed to loss of semen or semen-like substances. It ranges from somatic complaints, anxiety, weakness in the body, and masturbatory guilt associated with loss of vital fluid semen (Prakash 2007).

Though earlier considered only with males, what could be a female equivalent was reported as early as 1988 by Chaturvedi (Chaturvedi 1988). Female dhat syndrome is usually documented with the symptoms of aches and pains, headaches and poor concentration, which is attributed to the passage of white discharge in urine or from the vagina (Mehra et al. 2021; Grover et al. 2014).

M. S. Bhatia (✉)
Department of Psychiatry, UCMS & GTB Hospital, Delhi, India

A. Goyal
Department of Psychiatry, IHBAS, Delhi, India

© The Author(s), under exclusive license to Springer Nature Singapore Pte Ltd. 2024

S. K. Kar et al. (eds.), *Dhat Syndrome*,
https://doi.org/10.1007/978-981-99-8870-9_10

## 10.2 Myths and Misconceptions over Treatment

It is not uncommon when a young man of South East Asian descent who talks or discussing about sex as taboo in comparison to their Western counterpart to believe that semen loss due to night fall or excess masturbation is not healthy and causes weakness in the body. One of the reasons apart from the difficulty in discussing this freely is also related to the cultural beliefs of our society.

Hence, when they start feeling weakness which may be due to multiple other causes they attribute to semen loss. Furthermore, instead of consulting a mental health expert, they go to multiple doctors and even quacks for their solutions causing a delay in their treatment as well as possible side effects from different medicines which may have been given in the course of their treatment. Singh et al. in their study reported the mean duration of 1.85 ± 2.14 years of first visit for help seeking behavior and sometimes about 4.63 ± 5.3 to reach a mental health professional. This is more of an evidence that dhat syndrome patients at times follow a long path to a psychiatrist and may visit more than three health practitioners before (Singh et al. 2016).

Patients coming for treatment comes with an expectation of medicines or some supplements which can provide a solution to their problem and rejuvenate their sexuality and many times get disappointed when medicines are not prescribed (Grover et al. 2016a). In a study by Grover et al. in 2016 on treatment patterns, outcomes and reasons for drop out in Dhat syndrome of the 64 patients who were followed up at 6 months, only about one third were identified as those who completed their treatment, and rest were drop outs. Majority (42%) dropped out of treatment at later or end stages. Common reasons for dropout were: medications were not prescribed, there was no improvement, doesn't think it's a mental health problem or need to consult a mental health professional or not satisfied with treatment showing how the belief that treatment has to be with some medicine probably not from a mental health professional plays a key role in this disorder (Grover et al. 2016b). In a study by Bhatia and Malik (Bhatia and Malik 1991) it was reported that those on medications reported more improvement as compared to those on therapy not in line with the findings of Grover et al. Hence, the exploration of factors for the reason of drop out should be carefully evaluated before concluding.

## 10.3 Management of Dhat Syndrome

The mainstay of treatment of Dhat syndrome is Non-pharmacological including understanding an individual's knowledge and awareness, psycho-education and cognitive behavior therapy by addressing faulty beliefs. However, there are some situations where the role of medications or pharmacological treatment cannot be denied.

As is necessary in any clinical assessment, history taking plays a very crucial role. Complete and a detailed history is the key to making correct management goals. The history should not only include complaints reported by the patient and the chronology but also patient understanding of his own symptoms which will help in understanding of patient in holistic manner. History of chronic disease, comorbid diseases like diabetes, thyroid etc., neurological or trauma, use of any drugs like one prescribed routinely or over the counter medications, aphrodisiac drugs, prior surgeries and trauma should be enquired and documented. It should also include to evaluate for any issues related to sexual anatomy. Evidence of direct or indirect effects of alcohol and other recreational drugs like opioids. LSD, MDMA has been reported and same should be asked. Uses of such substances causes affect either to the anatomical, neurovascular or endocrine system by changing the levels of testosterone or prolactin (Avasthi et al. 2017). A careful general and physical examination should also be done before commencing any treatment. In case of women relevant gynecological examination can be done to rule out any infective etiology for white discharge and an appropriate management for the same can be instituted.

### *10.3.1 Pharmacological Approach*

On the basis of comorbid disorders or issues Dhat syndrome can be further categorized as (Avasthi and Nehra 2001).

1. Symptoms of Only Dhat syndrome - Patients explain the symptoms are due to semen loss; presenting symptoms – symptoms like hypochondriacal disorder, depression or anxiety disorders
2. Symptom of Dhat along with comorbid depressive and anxiety disorders- Dhat presented as an additional symptom
3. Dhat with comorbid sexual dysfunction

It is also postulated that Dhat may occur as primary and comorbidities like depression and anxiety may develop secondarily as a result of its impact on the psyche of the individual or vice versa. In either of these scenarios, a multicentric study by Grover et al. in 2015 reported that mental health comorbidities are in higher conjunction with Dhat syndrome (Grover et al. 2015).

It is reported that almost (51.3%) half of participants reported sexual dysfunction concluding it as one of the most common comorbidity with Dhat syndrome in this study. Premature ejaculation and erectile dysfunction were two commonly reported sexual dysfunction in this study group. Another school of thought also postulated that rather than a separate nosological entity, Dhat syndrome is an extension or a variation of presentation of Depression as per DSM criteria. It has been considered as an independent diagnosis however evidence for the same has been limited in longitudinal studies (Sameer et al. 2015). Apart from considerations for independent entity versus an expression of depression, it is also postulated to be a cultural variant of somatization disorders. Previous studies unlike the multicentric one reported depression to be more common with a prevalence between 40–66%. Features of hypochondriasis and high somatosensory amplification have been reported in Dhat syndrome without comorbidity. Symptoms of various psychiatric disorders have been found to be coexisting with that of Dhat syndrome. Some of the common disorders reported are somatoform and hypochondriacal disorders (approx. 40%), anxiety disorder in about 21–38%, 40% with premature ejaculation and erectile dysfunction in a study by Dhikav et al. Multiple other studies have reported other less common comorbidities like phobia, stress reactions, obsessive-compulsive disorders, body dysmorphic disorders, and delusional disorders (Deb and Balhara 2013) and even recurrent brief depressive disorder (Kar and Garg 2016).

### 10.3.2 Organic Association of Dhat Syndrome

The medical conditions e.g. Diabetes mellitus, Urinary Tract Infection (UTI), Renal Tuberculosis, Sexually Transmitted Diseases (including Human Immunodeficiency Virus), Chyluria, Fungal infections, Postsurgery, Malignancy, Lipiduria, Hyperoxaluria, Proteinuria, Excessive use of antacids and tonics (producing calciuria and phosphaturia), Alkalinity of urine, semen, dehydration etc. can produce turbidity in urine (Gulati et al. 2007; Vera et al. 2010). They need to be ruled out. Also, if present appropriate treatment can be provided with alkalinization of urine using syrup disodium hydrogen citrate, or antibiotics etc.

### 10.3.3 Dhat Alone

Each patient with Dhat syndrome reveals some unique characteristics as well as some specific health care needs and the clinician can tailor the treatment according to the needs of the person. Patients often expect energizing medications, revitalizing tonics, rejuvenating vitamins, and injections for their illness or something to improve their "man power" which has been lost due to loss of semen but get disappointed when not advised so. Though in cases only Dhat syndrome with no comorbidity, treatment mainly focuses on non-pharmacological methods in which some can benefit from antianxiety drugs, clonazepam, lorazepam etc. which can help in reducing anxiety and help in better psychological mindedness for non-pharmacological intervention.

### 10.3.4 Dhat Syndrome with Comorbid Depression and/ or Anxiety

As was earlier discussed that Dhat syndrome can be a variant of depression. It is because they have been known to share symptom profiles like weakness, fatigue, palpitations, and sleep disturbances. Accordingly, the treatments for Dhat syndrome can be the same as the treatments for depression. Bhatia and Malik have reported good results with them (Bhatia et al. 1989).

Selective Serotonin Reuptake Inhibitors like escitalopram, fluoxetine, and paroxetine are usually prescribed in patients with depression with good results and improvement in Dhat syndrome. Dhikav et al. reported the usefulness of these medicines and counselling in the management of Dhat syndrome with comorbid depression (Dhikav et al. 2008). Global improvement can be attributed at times to the improvement of depressive features alone. Paroxetine was seen as one of the most commonly prescribed antidepressants in patients with Dhat syndrome as was reported by Grover et al. 2016 (Grover et al. 2016b). However, one should be very careful that it is not a blanket treatment for all patients and one of the common side effects of the SSRI is sexual dysfunction or can be a part of depression per se, which on treatment can exaggerate the anxiety related to Dhat syndrome. In such scenarios, other antidepressants with less sexual side effects alternatives to SSRIs like bupropion, mirtazapine and newer drugs like vilazodone and vortioxetine can be considered for the treatment of depression (Jing and Straw-Wilson 2016).

At times, the patient may present with Dhat with depression and sexual dysfunction. In these cases, medicine can be selected after due consideration of comorbidities. On the other hand, paroxetine and fluoxetine have been commonly used in cases of premature ejaculation and can be useful in treating those with comorbid premature ejaculation.

### 10.3.5 Dhat with Sexual Dysfunction

In patients with Dhat syndrome and erectile dysfunction, apart from non-pharmacological treatments, pharmacological treatment like oral erectogenic vaso-active agents Phosphodiesterase inhibitor (PDE-5 inhibitors), i.e., sildenafil, tadalafil, vardenafil are now a days most commonly prescribed in cases of erectile dysfunction as first line drugs. They have shown efficacy and safety in men with erectile dysfunction. Apart from the efficacy they have also reported to have mild adverse effects and drop out treatment rates are similar to placebo. Among the available PDE-5 inhibitors, sildenafil and vardenafil have a short half-life, whereas tadalafil has a relatively longer half-life. The use of PDE 5 is contraindicated in those using nitrates and should not be prescribed. PDE 5 with antihypertensive medications or alpha-blockers can result in hypotension. Other drugs which can be used are Trazodone, Yohimibine, apomorphine, phentolamine, and L-arginine. Androgens as an adjunctive treatment also have been found useful in some patients with severe hypogonadism (Avasthi et al. 2017).

In pharmacological management of premature ejaculation following medications can be used;

- Topical anaesthetic agent like lignocaine, tricyclic antidepressants nortriptyline and Clomipramine with a recommended dose of 25–50 mg/day or 25 mg 4–24 h before intercourse;
- SSRI—Fluoxetine 5–20 mg/day; Paroxetine 10–40 mg/day, 3–4 hours before intercourse; Sertraline 25–200 mg or 50 mg 4–8 h before intercourse; Dapoxetine 30 and 60 mg, on demand use, 1–2 hours before intercourse;
- Tramadol–50 mg of tramadol oral dispersible tablets, and 100 mg of tramadol oral dispersible tablets, used on demand
- Topical therapies include Lidocaine/ prilocaine cream Lidocaine 2.5–5%, 20–30 min, before intercourse

Research has indicated that the use of PDE 5 and SSRI leads to better outcomes, than the first use of SSRI alone. Among the SSRIs, paroxetine and sertraline are found equally good, but paroxetine has been reported to be superior to fluoxetine, clomipramine and sertraline.

Almost more than three decades back, one study had studied treatment responses. Four groups with different treatments: an anxiolytic, an antidepressant, counseling, and a placebo pill were made. Though, the groups receiving any form of pharmacological intervention resulted in the greatest reduction of symptoms; the data may be skewed as the largest number of respondents who dropped out did so from the psychotherapy group (Bhatia et al. 1989).

A literature review conducted in 2015 suggested a three point trifurcation towards an integrated approach. As has been reported earlier that patients with Dhat syndrome take a long path to reach a mental health professional, probably an integration with other specialities and utilizing alternative medicine professionals can help in addressing these needs. First as psychiatry and psychology, managing the treatment aspects, second would be psychoeducation or improving awareness among other specialities (such as general medicine, dermatology, and urology) and last group of alternative medicine practitioners and traditional healers. This approach will help in reducing social stigma while still working through within cultural facets of the society (Kar and Sarkar 2015).

In some cases, placebos can be used for their treatment along with Cognitive Behavior Therapy. As depressive and anxiety disorders are common comorbidities observed in Dhat syndrome; hence, a trial of antidepressants and anxiolytic medications are considered to be useful in Dhat syndrome. The same has been acknowledged and accepted by other researchers too (Mehta et al. 2009). There are few case reports which have reported that distress due to excessive worry over semen loss can precipitate into a more serious mental illness and can present with prodromal symptoms of subthreshold positive, negative, mood, or cognitive symptoms before the onset of fully evolved a psychotic disorder. Epigenetic changes occurring due to semen loss anxiety resulted in Hypothalamic Pituitary Axis disruption are linked with its changeover to schizophrenia (Kar et al. 2016).

## 10.4 Current Research Status of Management and Future Directions Regarding the Management of Dhat Syndrome

Dhat syndrome has been discussed for more than six decades in multiple research articles specifically when catering to South east Asian countries. Its nosological status has received a place in ICD -10 as F48 under "other nonpsychotic mental disorders" (F48), DSM-5 quoted it in the "cultural concepts of distress" in the glossary making it more difficult to make a clear distinction in identification and management. Mumford has even contemplated Dhat syndrome as part of other psychiatric disorders. Studies have commented on presence of comorbidities or closely linked to depression and anxiety in patients with Dhat syndrome (Mumford 1996; Bhatia et al. 1989; Shakya 2019). The treatment discussion has since been encouraged in the management of these symptom profiles. As TSS Rao said in its discourse that this "cause-effect" dilemma can never be fully resolved. And barriers to successful treatment are due to frequent changes of physicians, irregular drug taking and irregular following the instructions, and high dropout from health care as the attributional beliefs persist even after repeated reassurance. (Sathyanarayana Rao 2004). The current concept on management focuses on a multimodal approach including mental health professionals like psychiatrists, clinical psychologists, and psychiatric social workers along with close liaison of the general physicians, the Ayurveda, Yoga, Unani, Siddha, Homeopathy practitioners, dermatologists and venereologists, and neurologists where patient may visit first due to his lack of awareness or denial of it being a mental health issue (Rao 2021). This liasioning will not only help in treating the organic causes but can also prevent overtreating any patient with Dhat syndrome. IPS Clinical practice guidelines for the management of sexual dysfunction can be looked upon for a detailed step-by-step process to assist in the management of patients presenting with Dhat syndrome and sexual dysfunction (Avasthi et al. 2017). No randomized trial or interventional studies have evaluated the effect of any intervention in these patients and primary evidence is available in the form of only observational or case studies (Kar et al. 2021). Evidence for treatment be it pharmacological, non-pharmacological or both with liaisons from various specialties can be strengthened by conducting randomized prospective studies.

## 10.5 Conclusion

Dhat syndrome has been discussed in its many forms from ancient scriptures to modern medicine. Management of Dhat syndrome encompasses detailed history taking, ruling out any medical or organic causes of white milky discharge, and assessment of knowledge and beliefs in the background of culture. The mainstay of treatment for Dhat syndrome is primarily non-pharmacological however antidepressants and antianxiety drugs have some usefulness in their treatment too. Careful evaluation of the presence of comorbid psychiatric disorders and sexual dysfunction and appropriate management can help in relieving symptoms at the earliest.

## References

Avasthi A, Grover S, Rao TS. Clinical practice guidelines for management of sexual dysfunction. Indian J Psychiatry. 2017;59(Suppl 1):S91.

Avasthi A, Nehra R. Sexual disorders: a review of Indian research. *Mental Health in India (1995–2000): People's Action for Mental Health*, 2001 42–53.

Bhatia MS, Bohra N, Malik SC. 'Dhat'syndrome—a useful clinical entity. Indian J Dermatol. 1989;34(2):32–41.

Bhatia MS, Malik SC. Dhat syndrome–a useful diagnostic entity in Indian culture. Br J Psychiatry. 1991;159(5):691–5.

Chaturvedi SK. Psychaesthenic syndrome related to leukorrhoea in Indian women. J Psychosom Obstet Gynecol. 1988;8(1):67–72.

Deb KS, Balhara YPS. Dhat syndrome: a review of the world literature. Indian J Psychol Med. 2013;35(4):326–31.

Dhikav V, Aggarwal N, Gupta S, Jadhavi R, Singh K. Depression in Dhat syndrome. J Sex Med. 2008;5(4):841–4.

Grover S, Avasthi A, Gupta S, Dan A, Neogi R, Behere PB, Lakdawala B, Tripathi A, Chakraborty K, Sinha V, Bhatia MS. Comorbidity in patients with Dhat syndrome: a nationwide multicentric study. J Sex Med. 2015;12(6):1398–401.

Grover S, Avasthi A, Gupta S, Dan A, Neogi R, Behere PB, Lakdawala B, Tripathi A, Chakraborty K, Sinha V, Bhatia MS. Phenomenology and beliefs of patients with Dhat syndrome: a nationwide multicentric study. Int J Soc Psychiatry. 2016a;62(1):57–66.

Grover S, Gupta S, Avasthi A. A follow-up study of patients with Dhat syndrome: treatment pattern, outcome, and reasons for dropout from treatment. Indian J Psychiatry. 2016b;58(1):49.

Grover S, Kate N, Avasthi A, Rajpal N, Umamaheswari V. Females too suffer from Dhat syndrome: a case series and revisit of the concept. Indian J Psychiatry. 2014;56(4):388.

Gulati S, Gupta N, Singh NP, Batra S, Garg S, Beniwal P, Kumar S. Chyluria with proteinuria or filarial nephropathy? An enigma. Parasitol Int. 2007;56(3):251–4.

Jing E, Straw-Wilson K. Sexual dysfunction in selective serotonin reuptake inhibitors (SSRIs) and potential solutions: a narrative literature review. Mental Health Clinician. 2016;6(4):191–6.

Kar SK, Garg K. Recurrent brief depressive disorder in Dhat syndrome: a biological or psychological phenomenon! Aust N Z J Psychiatry. 2016;50(3):291–2.

Kar SK, Menon V, Arafat SY, Singh A, Das A, Shankar A, Sharma P, Perera S. Dhat syndrome: systematic review of epidemiology, nosology, clinical features, and management strategies. Asian J Psychiatr. 2021;65:102863.

Kar SK, Sarkar S. Dhat syndrome: evolution of concept, current understanding, and need of an integrated approach. J Hum Reprod Sci. 2015;8(3):130.

Kar SK, Shahi MK, Tripathi A. Dhat syndrome as the prodrome of schizophrenia: understanding the cultural distress. Asian J Psychiatr. 2016;25:203–4.

Mehra A, Kathirvel S, Gainder S, Avasthi A, Grover S. Female Dhat syndrome in primary care setting. Ind Psychiatry J. 2021;30(2):278.

Mehta V, De A, Balachandran C. Dhat syndrome: a reappraisal. Indian J Dermatol. 2009;54(1):89.

Mumford DB. The 'Dhat syndrome': a culturally determined symptom of depression? Acta Psychiatr Scand. 1996;94(3):163–7.

Prakash O. Lessons for postgraduate trainees about Dhat syndrome. Indian J Psychiatry. 2007;49(3):208.

Rao TSS. Some thoughts on sexualities and research in India. Indian J Psychiatry. 2004;46(1):3.

Rao TSS. History and mystery of Dhat syndrome: a critical look at the current understanding and future directions. Indian J Psychiatry. 2021;63(4):317–25.

Sameer M, Menon V, Chandrasekaran R. Is 'Pure' Dhat syndrome a stable diagnostic entity? A naturalistic long term follow up study from a tertiary care Centre. J Clin Diagn Res. 2015;9(8):VC01–3.

Shakya DR. Dhat syndrome: study of clinical presentations in a teaching institute of eastern Nepal. J Psychosexual Health. 2019;1(2):143–8.

Singh A, Tripathi A, Gupta B, Agarwal V. Pathways to care for dhat (Semen loss anxiety) syndrome: a study from North India. Int J Ment Health. 2016;45(4):253–61.

Strong YN, Li A, White ME, Razzak AN, Anderson DJ, Kaye AD, Herron EW, Khater NP, Bradley EC, Urits I. Dhat syndrome: epidemiology, risk factors, comorbidities, diagnosis, treatment, and management. Health Psychol Res. 2022;10:4.

Vera M, Molano A, Rodríguez P. Turbid white urine. NDT Plus. 2010;3(1):45–7.

# Chapter 11
# Psychosocial Management of Dhat Syndrome

**Om Prakash and Shipra Singh**

## 11.1 Introduction

Dhat syndrome is a well-known culture-bound syndrome, which is characterized by excessive concern and preoccupation about loss of semen, vague somatic symptoms, fatigue, weakness and loss of appetite, prevalent across the Indian subcontinent, although similar conditions are not unknown in other parts of the world. Being a culture-bound syndrome, its origin lies in the belief system of a particular culture.

The term "*Dhat*" was adapted from the Vedic description of body fluids called "*Dhatus*", also called '*elixir*' or 'constituent part of the body'. Semen is perceived to be the most valuable among the seven different body fluids mentioned in Vedas (Prakash et al. 2014). Ancient Ayurveda literature also mentions genital secretions as highly precious and purified body fluid and emphasizes its conservation. The literature from Ayurveda unfolds the complex formation of semen through the process of purification involving multiple steps, thus making it extremely valuable (Prakash et al. 2014; Akhtar 1988). India is home to various religions and cultures, and it would be important to understand that many other religions, apart from Hinduism, share similar beliefs. In Islam, sexual dysfunction resulting from semen loss (Masturbation or prostitution), premature ejaculation, and impotency are described together as "*Mardana Kamzori*" (Hirsh 1996). On a related note, orthodox Christianity and Buddhism emphasized the sinful nature of masturbation and recognized the resulting semen loss as abnormal (Prakash et al. 2014). Semen, therefore, takes an overwhelmingly important role and any kind of loss or wastage of it was considered damaging to an individual's body.

---

O. Prakash (✉) · S. Singh
Department of Psychiatry, Institute of Human Behaviour and Allied Sciences (IHBAS), New Delhi, India

© The Author(s), under exclusive license to Springer Nature Singapore Pte Ltd. 2024

S. K. Kar et al. (eds.), *Dhat Syndrome*,
https://doi.org/10.1007/978-981-99-8870-9_11

Owing to the popular belief of the highly vital nature of semen, Dhat syndrome usually manifests as weakness, fatigue, palpitation, and insomnia, commonly seen in young, newly married males of low socio-economic status of rural background (Behere and Natraj 1984; Avasthi et al. 2008). It is often found associated with psychosexual disorders like erectile dysfunction and premature ejaculation as well as other psychiatric manifestations including depression, anxiety, pessimistic views of self and the future, etc., and attribute their symptoms to the passage of semen in urine or masturbation or sleep etc. (Grover et al. 2015).

Dhat syndrome has been linked to multiple factors; some of the more common ones of which are masturbation, unprotected sex, multiple sex partners and homosexual activity, erotic literature/movies, alcohol, straining at stools, drinking less water, less exercise, excess worry, nightfall, unnatural sex, 'excess heat in the body' (Prakash 2007; Prakash et al. 2014).

It is important to highlight that there have been a few studies about a comparable condition in females. These women describe vaginal discharge, which on examination, is non-pathological, not secondary to infection, and is associated with varied somatic and psychological symptoms. The symptoms are assumed secondary to the vaginal discharge, which is believed to be a vital fluid by many of them (Mehra et al. 2021).

## 11.2 Management

### *11.2.1 Assessment*

The assessment of Dhat syndrome typically involves a combination of clinical interviews, medical examinations, and psychological assessments (Prakash 2007; Avasthi et al. 2012). Step-wise approach for assessment is as follows:

(a) Clinical interview: Begin by conducting a thorough clinical interview with the individual experiencing the symptoms. This interview should focus on gathering information about the person's beliefs, symptoms, and concerns related to Dhat syndrome. It is important to approach the interview with cultural sensitivity and an open-minded attitude. Sexual history, including the beliefs about Dhat, physiological emissions, and sexual activity need to be explored in detail.

(b) Medical evaluation: Perform a comprehensive medical evaluation to rule out any underlying physical causes for the symptoms. This may involve conducting physical examinations, laboratory tests, and reviewing the person's medical history. It is crucial to identify and address any potential medical conditions that could be contributing to the symptoms.

(c) Psychological assessment: Assess the person's psychological well-being through standardized psychological assessments, such as questionnaires or interviews. This can help evaluate the person's mental health status, including symptoms of anxiety, depression, or obsessive-compulsive disorder, which are commonly associated with Dhat syndrome. A few questionnaires like the Comprehensive Questionnaire for Assessment of Dhat syndrome may be used for systematic assessment of such patients (Grover et al. 2014).

(d) Cultural understanding: It is important to gain an understanding of the person's cultural background and beliefs regarding Dhat syndrome. Also, recognize that cultural factors play a significant role in the manifestation and interpretation of symptoms. This understanding can help guide the assessment process and inform the treatment approach (Grover et al. 2014).

(e) Culturally sensitive approach: Throughout the assessment process, maintain a culturally sensitive approach and respect the person's beliefs and experiences. Engage in open and non-judgmental communication to create a safe environment for the individual to share their concerns (Grover et al. 2014).

### *11.2.2 Misconceptions Related to Dhat Syndrome*

Dhat syndrome has been recognized and studied within cultural contexts, there are several misconceptions surrounding Dhat syndrome (Manore et al. 2020; Prakash et al. 2018; Sawant and Nath 2012). One of the common misconceptions is that the perceived loss of semen in Dhat syndrome leads to physical and mental health issues. It is commonly believed that Dhat is a vital fluid, and is a source of power and energy. It is produced from a large quantity of blood, which after purification gets converted to Dhat. Its formation requires nutritious food. Loss of such valuable substance can cause various bodily problems like weakness, bodyache, headache, backache, mental symptoms like anxiety, lack of concentration, poor memory, and sexual problems like the small size of the penis, poor erection, early ejaculation, infertility etc. Frequent discharge of semen may affect physical health and may also cause thinning of semen and loss of vigor (Manore et al. 2020).

The other common myth remains that as semen is considered precious, therefore, it should not be wasted by masturbation. It is believed that masturbation may lead to physical and mental deterioration. Repetitive masturbation can lead to structural deformities like curving of the penis. Several myths and misconceptions are widely prevalent about penis in the society.

Myths also revolve around female Dhat syndrome (Mehra et al. 2021). Non-pathological white discharge per vagina, which is considered a vital fluid for the body, the loss of which lead to weakness, decrease in stamina, loss of physical beauty and may affect sexual health (loss of sexual desire, reduction in size of vagina/uterus, pain in genitals). It is also believed that mental health is affected as well and there may be an increased risk of malformation in children and more birth of female children to those suffering from this syndrome.

### *11.2.3 Differential Diagnoses*

While Dhat syndrome remains a distinct entity, clinicians must be aware of its potential differential diagnoses. Conducting a comprehensive evaluation, including a detailed psychiatric and medical history, physical examination, and appropriate laboratory investigations, can help differentiate Dhat syndrome from other conditions. Table 11.1 depicts some of the differentials of medical causes for the loss/leakage of semen (Roland 2018). Collaborative efforts between mental health professionals and physicians are essential in providing appropriate diagnosis and management to individuals presenting with symptoms suggestive of Dhat syndrome. If necessary, consult with specialists such as urologists, endocrinologists, psychiatrists, or psychologists who have experience working with Dhat syndrome or similar conditions. Collaborative efforts can provide a more comprehensive assessment and treatment plan. Ensure that the symptoms reported by the individual are not due to

**Table 11.1** Differential diagnoses of semen loss/leakage (Roland 2018)

| | What are other possibilities? | What else to look for? | What is important? |
|---|---|---|---|
| 1. | Side effects of medications (antidepressants, mood stabilizers, hormone treatments) | May be associated with other sexual side effects as well | Detailed treatment history |
| 2. | Prostate-related problems (Prostatitis, Prostate cancer) | Commonly associated with:<br>• Difficulty urinating<br>• Pain in the pelvic area<br>• Changes in ejaculation<br>• Blood in semen | Detailed medical history |
| 3. | Nerve injury (Advanced age, Infections, Injuries and surgery to the spinal cord or groin; exposure to poisons, e.g. carbon monoxide or heavy metals, degenerative conditions, e.g. Parkinson's disease, multiple sclerosis) | These may affect the nerves involved in ejaculation changes in ejaculation, leading to semen leakage | Detailed surgical and medical history |
| 4. | Medical conditions affecting nerves (Diabetes, Stroke; Degenerative conditions, such as Parkinson's disease, Multiple sclerosis; Nutritional deficiencies, such as a vitamin B-12; Guillain–Barré syndrome; Drug or alcohol misuse) | Changes in sexual function and ejaculation | Detailed neurological and medical history |
| 5. | Sexually transmitted infections | In cases, where the leaked fluid is discharged and not semen | Detailed sexual history |
| 6. | Retrograde ejaculation | Semen enters the bladder instead of exiting out of the penis, typically causing urine to be cloudy. | |

other conditions with similar presentations. It is important to differentiate Dhat syndrome from medical conditions or psychological disorders.

(a) Hypochondriasis: Hypochondriasis, also known as illness anxiety disorder, shares similarities with Dhat syndrome, particularly in terms of excessive preoccupation with bodily symptoms. Individuals with hypochondriasis have persistent fears of having a severe medical condition despite minimal or no medical evidence. Distinguishing features may include a broader focus on various bodily symptoms and concerns about general health rather than solely focusing on semen loss.
(b) Obsessive-Compulsive Disorder (OCD): OCD is a chronic psychiatric disorder characterized by intrusive thoughts (obsessions) and repetitive behaviours (compulsions). In some cases, individuals with OCD may experience obsessions related to contamination fears, including semen contamination. The main differentiating factor is the presence of obsessive thoughts and compulsive rituals aimed at preventing or reducing distress, which are absent in Dhat syndrome.
(c) Depression and Anxiety Disorders: Symptoms of depression and anxiety disorders, such as generalized anxiety disorder or social anxiety disorder, can sometimes overlap with Dhat syndrome. Psychological distress, including low mood, loss of interest, excessive worrying, and somatic complaints, may be present in both conditions. However, in depression and anxiety disorders, the symptoms are not limited to concerns about semen loss but encompass a broader range of emotional and cognitive symptoms.
(d) Somatoform Disorders: Somatoform disorders, particularly somatization disorder and conversion disorder, involve the manifestation of physical symptoms without an identifiable medical cause. These disorders can present with a wide array of somatic complaints, often spanning multiple organ systems. Dhat syndrome, on the other hand, tends to be more specific to concerns related to semen loss and associated symptoms.

## 11.3 Psychosocial Management

Psychosocial management is a crucial component in the comprehensive treatment of Dhat syndrome. By addressing the psychosocial aspects, healthcare professionals can improve the quality of life for individuals suffering from this syndrome. Psychoeducation, cognitive-behavioural therapy, relaxation techniques, psychosexual therapy, supportive counselling, and family involvement are all valuable interventions that can empower individuals and aid in their recovery. A multidimensional approach that combines medical, psychological, and sociocultural interventions can promote holistic healing and enhance the overall well-being of individuals with Dhat syndrome.

N.N. Wig suggested emphatic listening, a non - confrontational approach, reassurance and correction of erroneous beliefs, along with the use of placebo, anti-anxiety and antidepressant drugs, wherever required (Wig 1960). Avasthi and his colleagues proposed a management algorithm for Dhat syndrome (Avasthi et al. 2017).

### *11.3.1 Psychoeducation*

Psychoeducation is defined as "an intervention with systematic, structured, and didactic knowledge transfer for an illness and its treatment, integrating emotional and motivational aspects to enable patients to cope with the illness and to improve its treatment adherence and efficacy" (Ekhtiari et al. 2017). The initial step in psychosocial management is providing comprehensive psychoeducation to the individual and their family members. This involves imparting knowledge about the nature of Dhat syndrome, its cultural context, and the distinction between myths and medical facts. Educating the individual about the normal functioning of the body, reproductive system, and sexual health is essential to challenge misconceptions and reduce anxiety (Prakash and Kar 2019).

Individuals diagnosed with Dhat syndrome, tend to have very strong beliefs concerning semen's potency as a life force and the consequences of its loss. In addition, they consult to gain medications, which can revitalize them. In contrast, the management they expect is quite contradictory. Therefore, it is of utmost importance to have an empathetic, non-judgmental, non-confronting attitude while interacting with such patients. Psychoeducation in Dhat syndrome involves adequate sex knowledge and clarifying myths and misconceptions. Cultural sensitivity is of utmost importance when providing psychoeducation for Dhat syndrome. Understanding the cultural context and beliefs surrounding the syndrome is essential for effective communication and intervention. Sex education mainly focuses on the anatomy and physiology of sexual organs and their functioning concerning masturbation, semen formation, nocturnal emissions and their functioning with a genitourinary system independent of gastro-intestinal tract etc. (Prakash and Meena 2008; Hafi et al. 2022). Practitioners should be aware of cultural nuances, religious influences, and the impact of societal norms on the individual's perception and experience of Dhat syndrome. Taking a culturally sensitive approach ensures that interventions are tailored to the individual's background, beliefs, and values, promoting better engagement and treatment outcomes. Group sessions of psychoeducation may sometimes be considered, helping the participants to open up about their issues easily. The scope of psychoeducation becomes far wider, involving family members as well (Hafi et al. 2022). Psychoeducation in females suffering from the analogue of Dhat syndrome is nearly on similar lines as that of males, explaining the normal anatomy and physiology along with clarifying the myths (Tripathi et al. 2021).

Many interventions have combined psychoeducation/sex education with other modalities like cognitive behaviour therapy, relaxation exercise, medications, etc., although most of them remain unstructured and non-standardized.

### 11.3.2 Cognitive Behavior Therapy

Cognitive behaviour therapy (CBT) is a widely recognized therapeutic approach that has proven effective in treating Dhat syndrome. CBT can help individuals challenge and modify their cognitive distortions and dysfunctional beliefs related to semen loss. By identifying and addressing negative automatic thoughts, therapists can assist individuals in developing more adaptive coping strategies. Additionally, CBT can address co-occurring conditions such as anxiety and depression, which often accompany Dhat syndrome.

CBT is supposed to be a relevant intervention in Dhat syndrome because of faulty beliefs and misconceptions about the origin of their symptoms and sexual functioning. A sample cognitive model for Dhat syndrome can be understood in Fig. 11.1, adapted from the case study (Gupta 2017). A combination of psychoeducation and culturally informed cognitive behavioural therapy has also been suggested (Sumathipala et al. 2004). Tripathi and Sridevi mentioned interventions comprising of psychoeducation, supportive psychotherapy and CBT, which focused

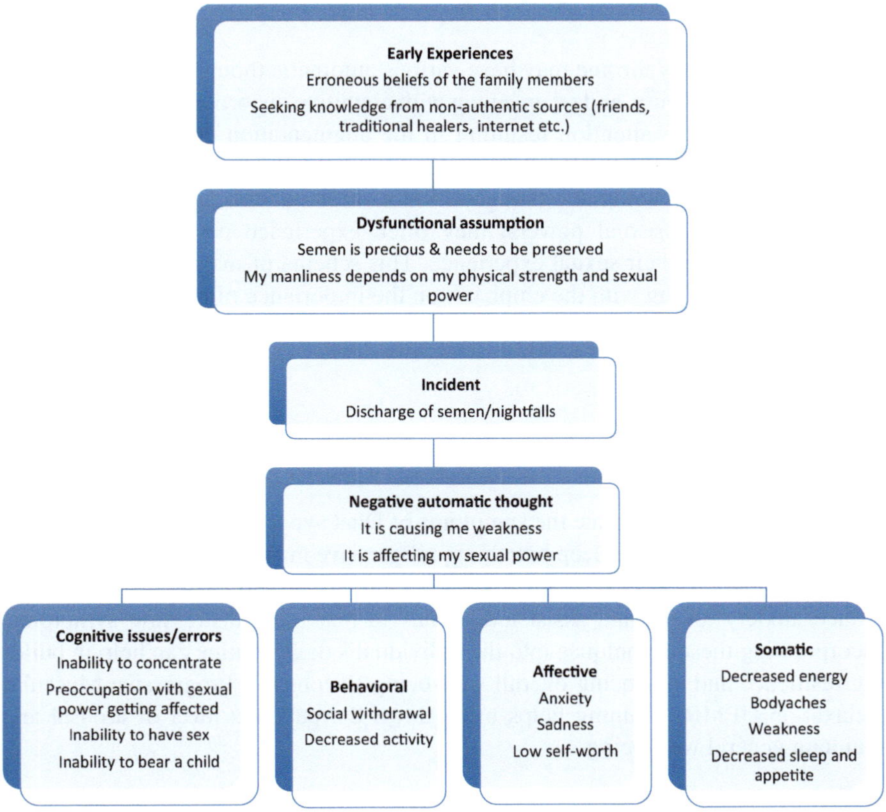


**Fig. 11.1** Cognitive model for Dhat syndrome (Gupta 2017)

on the catastrophizing automatic thought (or, in this case, the cultural belief) and cognitive techniques were used to restructure them. This intervention is compiled with activity scheduling, cognitive restructuring (thought challenging, role-playing, positive statements, and behavioural rehearsal and relaxation therapy (JPMR) (Tripathi and Sridevi 2014).

The first structured treatment program for Dhat Syndrome was developed by Salam and his colleagues. Their CBT module consisted of multiple components: sex education, cognitive restructuring, relaxation training, imaginal desensitization, masturbatory trainin', Kegel's exercises, 'start-stop technique' and 'squeeze technique' (in case of psychosexual disorders). It was found to be feasible in routine practice and was suitable for application within busy clinical settings (Salam et al. 2012). Some patients may find even the imagery of loss of semen as distressing, and therefore imaginal before actual (in vivo) desensitization (termed Imaginal desensitization), may be helpful in such cases. Masturbation as homework may help single males to better understand the harmlessness of loss of semen.

### *11.3.3 Cognitive Restructuring*

Patients with Dhat syndrome may have various automatic thoughts or beliefs about semen loss, masculinity, and so on, along with cognitive distortions like catastrophisation, and selective attention resulting in the augmentation and maintenance of somatic, sexual and other symptoms. The patient is encouraged to elicit alternative explanations for the automatic thoughts. Since these patients are immensely concerned about their sexual powers, they often experience performance anxiety, thereby hampering their sexual experience. This schema of masculinity also needs to be addressed, along with the emphasis on the importance of emotional and relationship factors in sexual relations.

### *11.3.4 Relaxation Techniques*

Stress and anxiety exacerbate the symptoms of Dhat syndrome. Therefore, teaching relaxation techniques like deep breathing, progressive muscle relaxation, and mindfulness meditation can be beneficial. These techniques promote a sense of calmness, reduce anxiety levels, and assist individuals in managing distressing symptoms. Incorporating these techniques into the individual's daily routine can help in building resilience and enhancing overall well-being. Jacobson's Progressive Muscular Relaxation (JPMR) Training helps bring down the patient's level of arousal and maintain general well-being.

### *11.3.5 Psychosexual Therapy*

Dhat syndrome is closely linked to sexual dysfunction and performance anxiety. Psychosexual therapy can be invaluable in addressing these concerns. Through open and non-judgmental communication, individuals can discuss their fears, anxieties, and misconceptions regarding sexual functioning. Psychosexual therapy aims to enhance sexual knowledge, promote healthy sexual attitudes, and provide practical techniques for overcoming sexual difficulties. This therapy can involve individual or couples counselling, depending on the needs of the person. In patients with associated psychosexual dysfunction, Kegel's exercises and other specific exercises like 'the squeeze technique' and 'the start-stop technique' are taught to the patient based on the specific problems.

### *11.3.6 Supportive Counselling*

Supportive counselling plays a crucial role in providing a safe and empathetic space for individuals to express their concerns, fears, and frustrations. The therapist can validate the individual's experiences, normalize their emotions, and offer guidance for coping with the challenges associated with Dhat syndrome. The therapeutic alliance formed during supportive counselling can be a source of comfort and encouragement throughout the treatment process.

### *11.3.7 Social Support and Family Involvement*

Social support is a crucial aspect of the psychosocial management of Dhat Syndrome. It plays a significant role in providing individuals with understanding, validation, and encouragement, as well as reducing feelings of isolation and stigma. Social support can come from various sources, including friends, family, peers, and support groups. In many cultures, family support and involvement are integral to an individual's well-being. Engaging the family members in therapy sessions can help them understand the nuances of Dhat syndrome and provide emotional support to the affected individual. Family members can also learn techniques to facilitate open communication, reduce stigma, and actively participate in the individual's recovery journey.

### 11.3.8 Support Groups

Support groups specifically tailored for individuals with Dhat Syndrome can be highly beneficial. These groups provide a safe and understanding environment where individuals can share their experiences, concerns, and challenges related to the syndrome. Being part of a support group helps individuals realize that they are not alone in their struggles, and it provides a platform for mutual support, information-sharing, and coping strategies.

### 11.3.9 Collaborative Care and Referral

An integrated 3-pronged approach is suggested to plan a comprehensive approach to the management of Dhat syndrome (Kar and Sarkar 2015). The first approach would be that a team consisting of psychiatrists, clinical psychologists and psychiatric social workers, along with specialists such as urologists or endocrinologists (who may be necessary to rule out any underlying physical conditions), work in unison, in the management of this syndrome. The second group is other medical disciplines (such as general medicine, dermatology, and urology) which are often approached by patients with Dhat syndrome before they have sought psychiatric help. These other specialities need education on the syndrome as well, so they know where to refer patients. Other physicians, who could encounter such patients in their practice, should also be educated to be empathetic and non-confronting, because as is already known that patients with Dhat syndrome have a poor follow-up rate and are known to frequently change physicians and even the system of medicine as well (Grover et al. 2016). Simultaneously, timely referral of such patients from other departments would lead to earlier initiation of treatment. The last group is alternative medicine practitioners and traditional healers. Working with this group will help combat the social stigma surrounding Dhat syndrome as well as help providers understand how to approach patient education in a culturally sensitive way.

### 11.3.10 Person-Centered Care

An emerging care model in psychiatric illnesses is person-centred care. Multiple factors may influence clinical decision-making including patients' characteristics, beliefs, and attitudes. These individuals often harbour culturally and socially driven myths about their symptoms. There is a need for individualized and holistic care programs for patients with Dhat syndrome considering their specific perceptions, experiences and interpretations of the symptoms. Person centred approach emphasizes giving due importance to the clinical characteristics, beliefs and opinions of the patient, preferences of the patients, and individual characteristics of the therapist as well as evidence-based management strategies (Kar and Singh 2016).

## 11.4 Conclusion

Dhat syndrome is a culturally bound syndrome primarily reported in South Asian countries, characterized by excessive concerns about semen loss through urine, leading to various somatic and psychological symptoms. The current modes of treatment that are found to be useful are reassurance, sex education, cognitive behavioural therapy, and counselling supplemented by medications (in specific cases), which help a proportion of men with these complaints, to improve. It is important to acknowledge the cultural significance and impact of the syndrome when working with individuals who report its symptoms. It is important to approach Dhat syndrome with cultural sensitivity and understanding, recognizing that its manifestations are influenced by cultural, psychological, and social factors. A comprehensive and holistic approach, involving psychological support, education, and addressing cultural beliefs, is crucial for individuals experiencing distress related to Dhat syndrome.

## References

Akhtar S. Four culture-bound psychiatric syndromes in India. Int J Soc Psychiatry. 1988;34:70–4.

Avasthi A, Grover S, Jhirwal OP. Dhat syndrome: a culture-bound sex related disorder in Indian subcontinent. In: Gupta S, Kumar B, editors. Sexually transmitted infections. 2nd ed. New Delhi, India: Elsevier; 2012. p. 1225–30.

Avasthi A, Grover S, Sathyanarayana Rao TS. Clinical practice guidelines for management of sexual dysfunction. Indian J Psychiatry. 2017;59:91–115.

Avasthi A, Kaur R, Prakash O, Banerjee A, Kumar L, Kulhara P. Sexual behavior of married young women: a preliminary study from North India. Indian J Community Med. 2008;33:163–7.

Behere PB, Natraj GS. Dhat syndrome: the phenomenology of a culture bound sex neurosis of the orient. Indian J Psychiatry. 1984;26:76–8.

Ekhtiari H, Rezapour T, Aupperle RL, Paulus MP. Neuroscience-informed psychoeducation for addiction medicine: a neurocognitive perspective. Prog Brain Res. 2017;235:239–64.

Grover S, Avasthi A, Aneja J, Shankar G, Mohan MR, Nehra R, Padhy SK. Comprehensive questionnaire for assessment of Dhat syndrome: development and use in patient population. J Sex Med. 2014;11(10):2485–95.

Grover S, Avasthi A, Gupta S, et al. Comorbidity in patients with Dhat syndrome: a nationwide multicentric study. J Sex Med. 2015;12(6):1398–401.

Grover S, Gupta S, Avasthi A. A follow-up study of patients with Dhat syndrome: treatment pattern, outcome, and reasons for dropout from treatment. Indian J Psychiatry. 2016;58(1):49–56.

Gupta P. Cognitive behaviour therapy for patients with Dhat syndrome: a case study. In: International conference on cognitive behavioural interventions—India 2017. New Delhi, India: AIIMS; 2017. p. 1–2.

Hafi B, Uvais NA, Varughese A, Aysha S. Dhat syndrome by proxy: an underreported entity. Primary Care Companion CNS Disord. 2022;24(2):40648.

Hirsh A. Post-coital sperm retrieval could lead to the wider approval of assisted conception by some religions. Hum Reprod. 1996;11:245–7.

Kar S, Sarkar S. Dhat syndrome: evolution of concept, current understanding, and need of an integrated approach. J Hum Reprod Sci. 2015;8(3):130–4.

Kar SK, Singh A. Person centered management approach for the Dhat syndrome. Int J Pers Cent Med. 2016;6(4):298–304.

Manore S, Vankar GK, Gedam S. Dhat syndrome: depression, help-seeking and patient beliefs about causation and consequences. Int J Curr Res Rev. 2020;12(21):123.

Mehra A, Kathirvel S, Gainder S, Avasthi A, Grover S. Female Dhat syndrome in primary care setting. Indian J Psychiatry. 2021;30(2):278–84. https://doi.org/10.4103/ipj.ipj_76_20.

Prakash O. Lessons for postgraduate trainees about Dhat syndrome. Indian J Psychiatry. 2007;49:208–10.

Prakash O, Kar SK. Dhat syndrome: a review and update. J Psychosexual Health. 2019;1(3–4):241–5.

Prakash O, Kar SK, Sathyanarayana Rao TS. Indian story on semen loss and related Dhat syndrome. Indian J Psychiatry. 2014;56:377–82.

Prakash O, Meena K. Association between Dhat and loss of energy—a possible psychopathology and psychotherapy. Med Hypotheses. 2008;70(4):898–9.

Prakash S, Sharan P, Sood M. A qualitative study on psychopathology of dhat syndrome in men: implications for classification of disorders. Asian J Psychiatr. 2018;35:79–88.

Roland J. What causes semen leakage and how to treat it. Sex Health. 2018; https://www.healthline.com/health/mens-health/semen-leakage

Salam KPA, Sharma MP, Prakash O. Development of cognitive-behavioral therapy intervention for patients with Dhat syndrome. Indian J Psychiatry. 2012;54(4):367–74.

Sawant N, Nath A. Cultural misconceptions and associated depression in Dhat syndrome. Sri Lanka J Psychiatry. 2012;3:1.

Sumathipala A, Siribaddana SH, Bhugra D. Culture-bound syndromes: the story of dhat syndrome. Br J Psychiatry. 2004;184:200–9.

Tripathi A, Roy D, Kar SK. Distress due to nonpathological vaginal discharge: a new face of Dhat syndrome in females. J Psychosexual Health. 2021;3(4):315–21.

Tripathi M, Sridevi G. CBT in Dhat syndrome and co-morbid conditions. Int J Sci Res Publ. 2014;4(9):1–8.

Wig NN. Problem of mental health in India. J Clin Soc Psychiatry. 1960;17:48–53.

# Chapter 12
# Female Dhat Syndrome

**Pawan Sharma, Swarndeep Singh, and Arghya Pal**

## 12.1 Introduction

Culture-bound syndromes represent a group of disorders that are still evolving in terms of their phenomenological and ontological status (Sumathipala et al. 2004). Dhat syndrome is arguably one of the most researched diagnostic entities from the South- East Asian region. It is speculated that the prevalence of Dhat syndrome is higher in the countries falling in the South-East Asian region. To some extent that is also substantiated by the higher volume of research on Dhat syndrome coming from these countries. But culture-bound syndromes are known for their knack of being difficult to be defined and to be tamed within the rigours of a diagnostic framework. Dhat syndrome has also been fraught with similar issues. Despite reasonable attempts, a consensus on the definition of Dhat Syndrome is still out of reach. To conceptualize it as a multimodal disorder with an overlap of anxiety, depressive, sexual, and psychosomatic phenomenology has been the most popular opinion, but even this approach does not provide insight into the whole conundrum. Initially, it was also presumed that Dhat syndrome is probably a geographically localized phenomenon, but that has been refuted by the increasing number of cases reported from various regions of the world like China, Japan, Russia, and several European countries (Rao 2021). To add to the challenge, researchers also started to realize that

P. Sharma (✉)
Department of Psychiatry, Patan Academy of Health Sciences, School of Medicine, Lalitpur, Nepal

S. Singh
Department of Psychiatry, Vardhman Mahavir Medical College & Safdarjung Hospital, Delhi, India

A. Pal
Department of Psychiatry, All India Institute of Medical Sciences, Raebareli, Uttar Pradesh, India

© The Author(s), under exclusive license to Springer Nature Singapore Pte Ltd. 2024

S. K. Kar et al. (eds.), *Dhat Syndrome*,
https://doi.org/10.1007/978-981-99-8870-9_12

females also present with complaints that are very similar to Dhat Syndrome, though most of the initial literature postulated it to be a condition affecting exclusively males.

But by the start of the 1990s, clinicians started reporting female patients that had stark phenomenological similarities with male patients of Dhat syndrome. These patients presented with multiple somatic symptoms like easy fatigability, vague pain symptoms and irritability with an overlay of depressive and anxiety symptoms. The women tended to pathologically attribute the symptoms to the discharge of fluid from the vagina. Such patients also ignited the effects of socio-cultural beliefs on various aspects of health (including mental health) and thus the search for female Dhat syndrome began among the research fraternity.

## 12.2 History of Female Dhat Syndrome

Etymologically the term 'Dhat Syndrome' has been derived from the word '*dhatu*', which if translated in *Sanskrit* means metal. Essentially, the phenomenological explanation of Dhat Syndrome in males is derived from the concept mentioned in *Charak Samhita*, a very similar presentation was also observed amongst females (Mehta et al. 2009). In the cases of females, the vital fluid that they were concerned with was whitish vaginal discharge. This whitish vaginal discharge has complex cultural underpinning. It is postulated in Ayurveda that whitish discharge of the vagina is indicative of a grave health condition with a poor prognosis ranging from various kinds of infections to incurable cancers. It is believed that these disorders may be associated with overheating in the body which leads to the dissolution of essential elements of the body and finally leaks out in the form of vaginal discharge.

The reports of females suffering from Dhat syndrome started surfacing around the late 1980s when Chaturvedi reported neurasthenic symptoms appearing in a female with a conservative upbringing attributing the symptoms to vaginal discharge (Chaturvedi 1988). Subsequently, other studies were also published that linked various forms of somatic symptoms to the discharge of the vaginal fluid (Rao 2021; Chaturvedi et al. 1993; Singh et al. 2001).

## 12.3 Nosological Evolution of Female Dhat Syndrome

However, though this rising number of articles endorsed the existence of female Dhat Syndrome, the approach of the various classificatory systems followed a different viewpoint. The tenth Edition of the *International Classification of Diseases (ICD 10)* mentioned Dhat Syndrome under the 'Other specified neurotic disorders' diagnostic category. The contemporary text revision of the fourth edition of the *Diagnostic and Statistical Manual of Mental Disorders* (DSM IV-TR) had also listed Dhat Syndrome as a culture-bound syndrome under the heading of "locality-specific patterns of aberrant behaviour, recurrent, and troubling experience, that may or may not be linked to a particular DSM-IV diagnostic category indigenously considered to be illnesses, or at least afflictions". Despite this, the debate went on regarding its position as a separate diagnostic entity even after this as dhat syndrome was considered a variant of depression or somatization disorder due to its comorbidity and the symptom profile (Arafat 2017). One school of thought is that the explanation of semen loss as fluid is a cultural idiom of distress rather than a standalone diagnostic entity and a pure form of Dhat syndrome doesn't have considerable diagnostic stability (Sameer et al. 2015). Another school considers Dhat syndrome a global phenomenon, rather than a culture-bound syndrome (Kar 2015). The DSM 5 has considerably deviated from this viewpoint and they have completely removed the section of 'culture-bound syndrome'. It has been replaced by the new entity called cultural concepts of distress.' This includes three sub-concepts—syndromes, idioms, and explanations; which will be used to understand the various maladaptive thoughts and emotions. Importantly, ICD 11 conspicuously has been silent about the diagnostic status of Dhat syndrome. From the perspective of female dhat syndrome though, the approach of ICD 11 is hindering, because most of the available research conducted on this topic has stressed on the fact that it would be beneficial for the sake of clinical practice to adopt female dhat syndrome as a valid diagnostic entity (Tripathi et al. 2021).

## 12.4 Epidemiology of Female Dhat Syndrome

Considering the ongoing discussion on the validity of female Dhat syndrome and the limited literature, there is an understandable dearth of epidemiological studies. Dhat syndrome in females has been reported in the literature in the form of case reports and case series, especially from India (Singh et al. 2001) Grover et al. 2014); Kar and Singh 2017). There is a common notion that the prevalence of Dhat syndrome in females is significantly lesser than that seen in males (Shakya 2019). In a study among 70 consecutive females of the reproductive age group presenting with multiple psychosomatic complaints, it was seen that 40% of females complained about vaginal discharge and 32% of them attributed their somatic symptoms to vaginal discharge (Chaturvedi 1988). A house-to-house survey among 236 married women aged 15–45 years from rural north India suggested a prevalence of vaginal discharge to be about 28.7%. The main health effects of vaginal discharge as reported by the females were weakness, backache and poor vision; and they believed excessive body heat, melting of bones, sexual promiscuity, poor hygiene and dietary factors as the major causes of vaginal discharge (Singh 2007). A community-based survey of 2494 women aged 18–50 years found that 14.5% had complaints of having an abnormal vaginal discharge, and stress was revealed as the most common causal attribution upon detailed assessment including laboratory testing and psychosocial evaluation (Patel et al. 2005).

## 12.5 Comparison with Dhat Syndrome Between Males and Females

Though female Dhat syndrome is a phenomenon that has many core similarities with the male Dhat syndrome, there are some notable differences as well. The mean age of onset is likely to be higher for females as compared to males i.e. 36.1 years vs. 24 years (Mehra et al. 2021) Bhatia et al. 1989). The reasons for female Dhat syndrome also differ from males. A study in primary care setting from India among 69 females having non-pathological vaginal discharge showed that the reasons reported for their discharge were consumption of warm foods and drinks (75.8%), followed by eating unbalanced/ inappropriate food (73.5%). They also reported other reasons like stress and emotional factors, infection, and the effect of warm weather leading to excess heat in the body (Mehra et al. 2021). Most patients thought their vaginal discharge was responsible for bodily weakness, backache, and stomach ache. These are similar to the presentation in males where they show symptoms of weakness, guilt, lethargy, anxiety, loss of appetite, sleep disturbances, listlessness, lack of physical strength, poor concentration, forgetfulness, multiple body pains, sexual dysfunction, burning micturition, increased frequency of micturition, difficulty in micturition (Arafat 2017). A significant proportion of females believe they are losing a vital fluid of the body similar to that of males. There is definite merit in considering the female equivalent of Dhat syndrome similar to the syndrome reported in males. The case for this becomes further strengthened, when we compare the clinical description of cases of non-infectious vaginal discharge with findings in male patients of Dhat syndrome (Grover et al. 2014).

## 12.6 Assessment of Female Dhat Syndrome

Vaginal discharge is the second most common presenting gynaecological complaint following menstrual cycle-related problems among treatment-seeking women. Further, when women in the reproductive age group from South Asia presenting with complaints of vaginal discharge were evaluated for psychosocial, infective and other common non-infective causes; about one-third to half of them were diagnosed to have non-pathological vaginal discharge (Tripathi et al. 2021). Non-pathological vaginal discharge (see Box 12.1) or leukorrhea is the cardinal feature in women with female Dhat Syndrome. This is also referred to as *safed paani* (whitish liquid), dhat/ dhatu (vital fluid), or *swed pradhar* (whitish discharge) by women. All women presenting with this complaint should be evaluated for the possibility of female Dhat Syndrome through careful history, clinical examination, and relevant lab investigations. The operational criteria that have been proposed for making the diagnosis of female Dhat Syndrome are as follows (Grover et al. 2014)

- Presence of non-pathological vaginal discharge (whitish, odourless vaginal discharge; local examination and/or laboratory findings not suggestive of any pathology)
- Persistent preoccupation/ marked worry or distress about the loss of genital secretions through this vaginal discharge
- Presence of multiple often vague physical or somatic symptoms (e.g., body aches, weakness); mental and psychological symptoms such as loss of interest, low mood, excessive worry or anxiety related to vaginal discharge (Note: Depending upon the nature and severity of these symptoms patients may also have another co-morbid psychiatric diagnosis such as depression)
- Attribution of these somatic and/or mental symptoms to the passage of vaginal discharge

However, due to the taboo associated with discussing sexual topics and the high levels of embarrassment experienced by women in most South-Asian societies about expressing this complaint (i.e. vaginal discharge) to healthcare professionals, diagnosing female Dhat Syndrome may be difficult at times. Subsequently, many times women present with either physical/ somatic complaints and/ or anxiety or excessive worry related to the loss of genital secretions in the form of vaginal discharge after a prolonged period (in years) of onset of leukorrhea. Thus, female is likely to be underdiagnosed or misdiagnosed by healthcare professionals during initial assessments (Sim et al. 2020). Table 12.1 summarizes the different types of physical, psychological, and sexual problems women with female Dhat Syndrome may report during the clinical encounter. A high index of clinical suspicion is necessary for recognizing women who might be suffering from female Dhat Syndrome when one complains of commonly associated vague and multiple somatic symptoms listed in Table 12.1 that are not being better explained by any other medical condition (e.g., urinary or reproductive tract infection).

Standardized assessment tools may also be used for making a further enquiry about other associated symptoms among women with female Dhat Syndrome. The two most commonly used assessment tools are described below:

***Scale for Assessment of Female Dhat Syndrome (SAFeD)*** This self-report-based instrument has been developed by modifying the "Dhat Syndrome Questionnaire" designed for a comprehensive assessment of male Dhat syndrome (Grover and

**Table 12.1** Common symptoms reported among women with Female Dhat Syndrome

| | |
|---|---|
| Physical/Somatic symptoms | Burning sensation or tingling in hands and/or feet, Weakness or excessive tiredness, Dizziness, Backache, Stomach ache, Joint pain, Visual symptoms like eye pain or weakness of eyesight, Lower abdominal pain unrelated to menses |
| Psychological symptoms | Depressive and anxiety symptoms, Irritability, Poor attention and concentration, Sleep disturbances |
| Sexual dysfunction symptoms | Loss of libido, Anorgasmia, Painful sexual intercourse, Sexual weakness |

Shouan 2020). It helps the interviewer to assess and establish the clinical criteria of female Dhat syndrome such as characteristics of dhat (e.g. duration, amount, colour, consistency, odour, and nature of vaginal discharge), associated physical/ somatic symptoms, and its psychological impact. It also explores personal beliefs held by the women about the perceived causes and perceived complications from loss of genital secretions or dhat in the form of vaginal discharge and assesses their perceived need for treatment and help-seeking beliefs including perceived effectiveness of different pharmacological and non-pharmacological treatment strategies for female Dhat Syndrome.

***Female Sexual Function Index (FSFI)*** The scale consists of 19 self-rated questions on a five-point Likert scale, and it has been used to measure sexual functioning among women (Grover and Shouan 2020). It assesses the following six domains of female sexual functioning: desire (2 questions), arousal (4 questions), lubrication (4 questions), orgasm (3 questions), satisfaction (3 questions), and pain (3 questions). Higher scores are indicative of better functioning, and cut-off scores have been recommended by researchers for diagnosing female sexual dysfunction in the past one-month period. This scale has been translated into several different languages including Hindi. Thus, it might be a useful adjunctive tool to assist clinicians in systematically evaluating sexual functioning and associated comorbid sexual dysfunctions among women with female Dhat syndrome.

## 12.7 Treatment of Female Dhat Syndrome

Once the diagnosis of female Dhat Syndrome has been established after ruling out possible medical causes of vaginal discharge. It is important to screen all these women for any other commonly found comorbid physical (e.g., anaemia, hypothyroidism) and/ or psychiatric disorders such as depression, anxiety disorders. Also, there is a need to build rapport with the women and reassure them that their symptoms are real and are being taken seriously by the treating clinician or team. This helps in making the women comfortable and improves their acceptance of the management provided by the treating team. Although, no standard treatment guidelines have yet been developed for female Dhat Syndrome. The available evidence from published case reports or case series, and the authors' own clinical experience of successfully managing women with female Dhat Syndrome suggests that the best results are obtained with a combination of psychological and pharmacological treatment strategies (Tripathi et al. 2021).

### 12.7.1 Psychological Therapy

A genuine attempt to explore and understand the associated beliefs held by women about the causal models behind the female dhat syndrome should be made by the health care professionals. For example, often there is a prevalent belief among women with female Dhat Syndrome that genital secretions comprise of vital fluid (e.g., 100 drops of blood make a single drop of *safed panni*) or vaginal discharge is a result of some internal disease or hollowing of bones or manifestation of excessive heat inside the body; and its loss from the body would result in weakness or other serious health problems. These faulty beliefs are a result of poor knowledge about the female reproductive system and physiology, along with reinforcement of these beliefs by other trustworthy people around them (e.g., mother, elder sister, friend) or local traditional healers (e.g., Ayurvedic practitioner) who are often the first point of contact for seeking help about health-related matters.

Interestingly, a study among 26 women with female Dhat Syndrome seeking treatment at a tertiary care hospital in North India reported that about 42% of them believed that treatment with energizing medications like multivitamins or tonics would be effective in relieving their symptoms (Grover et al. 2016). Whereas, only about 15% of them believed that counselling by a doctor would be an effective treatment for their complaints. Thus, expressing empathy and acknowledging their concerns related to the loss of genital secretions is important to initially build rapport with these women. This should be followed by psychoeducation sessions in which the women should be provided with correct sexual knowledge including information related to the anatomy of the male and female reproductive system (models or charts may be used), production of normal physiological vaginal discharge, its intended purpose, different conditions or factors that may result in increased non-pathological vaginal discharge in women, and any other myths associated with vaginal discharge should be addressed. Additionally, if required supportive psychotherapy or relaxation exercises can also be used to reduce the distress or excessive worry associated with loss of genital secretions in women with female Dhat Syndrome. Cognitive behaviour therapy to correct faulty beliefs about vaginal discharge, and minimize emotional distress symptoms associated with loss of genital secretions and/ or other psychosocial stressors should also be considered for women not responding adequately with supportive psychotherapy and psychoeducation sessions.

### 12.7.2 Pharmacological Therapy

The co-morbid physical or psychiatric disorders often detected among women with female Dhat Syndrome must be adequately treated. For example, depression or anxiety disorder symptoms should be treated by starting selective serotonin reuptake inhibitors (e.g., fluoxetine, escitalopram) or other atypical antidepressants with more favourable sexual side effect profiles (e.g., bupropion, mirtazapine) in doses as recommended for treatment of depression or specific anxiety disorder. Further, if severe anxiety symptoms or significant sleep disturbances occur in female Dhat Syndrome; benzodiazepines may be prescribed on a need basis or a short course of a few weeks under the guidance of a psychiatrist.

Kar and Sarkar suggest a need for an integrated approach where the following could be done (Kar and Sarkar 2015):

- Integration of psychiatry and allied disciplines (the collaborative approach of psychiatrists, psychologists, psychiatric social workers, psychiatric nurses, etc.)
- Integration of other medical disciplines with psychiatry (collaborative approach with other medical disciplines such as—general medicine, dermatology and venereology, urology, gynaecology and neurology)
- Integration with alternative systems of medicine and traditional healers (collaboration with Ayurvedic, Homeopathic, Unnani, Siddha practitioners).

**Box 12.1 Non-Pathological (or Normal Physiological) Vaginal Discharge**

**Characteristics:** Normal physiological vaginal discharge is made up of mucoid secretions released by endocervical glands lining the cervix, normally sloughed-off epithelial cells of the vagina and vaginal transudate. The amount of this non-pathological vaginal discharge (NPVD) varies during different phases of the menstrual cycle, and on average ranges between 1–4 ml of fluid per 24 h. NPVD is usually whitish or transparent in colour, with variable consistency ranging from thick and slightly yellowish during luteal phase to watery and stretchable around the time of ovulation, and mostly odourless or slightly malodorous (due to mixing with sweat). It serves to provide lubrication of the vagina and provides an acidic pH (4.0–4.5) that limits the growth of harmful bacteria in the vagina

**Absence of additional symptoms:** NPVD is usually not accompanied by any other symptoms often associated with infectious or inflammatory pathologies. These additional symptoms include: Any marked change in volume (e.g. excessive secretion), colour (e.g. reddish or dark yellow), or odour (e.g. fishy odour) of vaginal discharge, pruritus, significant burning sensation or irritation in the vagina, erythema (redness) or local erosions of the vagina, or spotting/ non-menstrual bleeding from the vagina. The absence of these signs and symptoms helps distinguish NPVD from discharge related to some underlying pathological condition (e.g., vaginitis, genital cancer, etc.)

**Factors affecting vaginal discharge:** Normal physiological vaginal discharge changes with different phases of the menstrual cycle as explained above. It may become more noticeable in women around the middle of the menstrual cycle close to the time of ovulation or during pregnancy. Vaginal discharge may also increase without any pathology during high estrogen states produced due to oral contraceptive use or hormone replacement therapy. Additionally, certain dietary habits, patterns of sexual activity, and emotional stress levels may also affect the volume and character of vaginal discharge in a non-harmful manner

## 12.8 Recommendations

There have been studies focused on female Dhat syndrome in the context of South East Asia especially India, but there remains much to be understood about the condition. As seen in the male Dhat syndrome, the diagnostic criteria for female Dhat syndrome remain ambiguous. However, there is no denying the fact that there is a deep cultural meaning behind this condition. We must understand it better to manage it more effectively. Therefore, we recommend qualitative studies on the phenomenology and development of effective scales for female Dhat syndrome. The concept of Dhat syndrome has been described as the "neurosis of the Orient" but this has been described historically in other cultures, including Britain, the USA and Australia suggesting the symptoms are universal and prevalence is global (Sumathipala et al. 2004). Hence there is a need to explore the female Dhat syndrome in other cultures as well.

## 12.9 Conclusion

Dhat syndrome in the female has a definite clinical utility and diagnostic relevance; and is comparable to male Dhat Syndrome in several aspects. However, there is ambiguity in some aspects like diagnostic criteria, epidemiology and its position in classificatory system. As it is an underdiagnosed entity, a comprehensive evaluation of non-pathological vaginal discharge is needed. A proper understanding of this entity would help in development of integrated approach for its management.

## References

Arafat SY. Dhat syndrome: culture bound, separate entity, or removed. J Behav Health. 2017;6(3):147–50. https://doi.org/10.5455/jbh.20170123102726.

Bhatia MS, Bohra N, Malik SC. "Dhat" syndrome—a useful clinical entity. Indian J Dermatol. 1989;34(2):32–41.

Chaturvedi SK. Psychaesthenic syndrome related to leukorrhoea in Indian women. J Psychosom Obstet Gynecol. 1988;8(1):67–72. https://doi.org/10.3109/01674828809016782.

Chaturvedi SK, Chandra PS, Isaac MK, Sudarshan CY, et al. Is there a female dhat syndrome? NIMHANS J. 1993;11:89–93.

Grover S, Avasthi A, Gupta S, Hazari N, Malhotra N. Do female patients with nonpathological vaginal discharge need the same evaluation as for Dhat syndrome in males? Indian J Psychiatry. 2016;58(1):61–9. https://doi.org/10.4103/0019-5545.174376.

Grover S, Kate N, Avasthi A, Rajpal N, Umamaheswari V. Females too suffer from Dhat syndrome: a case series and revisit of the concept. Indian J Psychiatry. 2014;56(4):388–92. https://doi.org/10.4103/0019-5545.146537.

Grover S, Shouan A. Assessment scales for sexual disorders—a review. J Psychosexual Health. 2020;2(2):121–38. https://doi.org/10.1177/2631831820919581.

Kar SK. Dhat syndrome: will it reach a height or die soon? J Hum Reprod Sci. 2015;8(4):246. https://doi.org/10.4103/0974-1208.170421.

Kar SK, Sarkar S. Dhat syndrome: evolution of concept, current understanding, and need of an integrated approach. J Hum Reprod Sci. 2015;8(3):130–4. https://doi.org/10.4103/0974-1208.165143.

Kar SK, Singh A. Where lies the fault in diagnosing Dhat syndrome among females? Understanding through a case study. Indian J Psychol Med. 2017;39(4):506–8. https://doi.org/10.4103/0253-7176.211742.

Mehra A, Kathirvel S, Gainder S, Avasthi A, Grover S. Female Dhat syndrome in primary care setting. Ind Psychiatry J. 2021;30(2):278–84. https://doi.org/10.4103/ipj.ipj_76_20.

Mehta V, De A, Balachandran C. Dhat syndrome: a reappraisal. Indian J Dermatol. 2009;54(1):89–90. https://doi.org/10.4103/0019-5154.49002.

Patel V, Pednekar S, Weiss H, Rodrigues M, Barros P, Nayak B, et al. Why do women complain of vaginal discharge? A population survey of infectious and pyschosocial risk factors in a South Asian community. Int J Epidemiol. 2005;34(4):853–62. https://doi.org/10.1093/ije/dyi072.

Rao TSS. History and mystery of Dhat syndrome: a critical look at the current understanding and future directions. Indian J Psychiatry. 2021;63(4):317–25. https://doi.org/10.4103/psychiatry.IndianJPsychiatry_791_20.

Sameer M, Menon V, Chandrasekaran R. Is 'pure' Dhat syndrome a stable diagnostic entity? A naturalistic long term follow up study from a tertiary care Centre. J Clin Diagn Res. 2015;9(8):VC01–3. https://doi.org/10.7860/JCDR/2015/13399.6275.

Shakya DR. Dhat syndrome: study of clinical presentations in a teaching institute of eastern Nepal. J Psychosexual Health. 2019;1(2):143–8. https://doi.org/10.1177/2631831819853742.

Sim M, Logan S, Goh LH. Vaginal discharge: evaluation and management in primary care. Singap Med J. 2020;61(6):297–301. https://doi.org/10.11622/smedj.2020088.

Singh AJ. Vaginal discharge: its causes and associated symptoms as perceived by rural north Indian women. Indian J Community Med. 2007;32(1):22. https://doi.org/10.4103/0970-0218.53388.

Singh G, Avasthi A, Pravin D. Dhat syndrome in a female- a case report. Indian J Psychiatry. 2001;43(4):345–8.

Sumathipala A, Siribaddana SH, Bhugra D. Culture-bound syndromes: the story of dhat syndrome. Br J Psychiatry J Ment Sci. 2004;184:200–9. https://doi.org/10.1192/bjp.184.3.200.

Tripathi A, Roy D, Kar SK. Distress due to nonpathological vaginal discharge: a new face of Dhat syndrome in females. J Psychosexual Health. 2021;3(4):315–21. https://doi.org/10.1177/26318318211049547.

# Chapter 13
# Public Health Aspects of Dhat Syndrome

**Russell Kabir, Madhini Sivasubramanian, Sumayea Binte Mizan, and Ali Davod Parsa**

## 13.1 Introduction

Dhat syndrome is a culture-bound psychiatric syndrome predominantly reported in Indian subcontinent countries such as India, Bangladesh, and Pakistan (Prakash et al. 2014). Dhat syndrome men perceived semen ejaculation as a loss of a precious substance that caused them to experience physical and psychological disorders and sexual problems (Prakash 2007). Rooted from the Sanskrit language word 'Dhat' or dhatu, meaning 'metal,' 'elixir' or 'essential part of the body', 'the most concentrated, perfect and powerful bodily substance that its preservation secures health and longevity (Prakash and Kar 2019). Some cultures value sperm highly and consider it to be a precious resource. Losing sperm is related to sexual problems and physical and mental illnesses. Dhat syndrome (Avasthi and Nehra 2001) triggers sexual dysfunction (Behere and Natraj 1984; De Silva and Dissanayake 1989; Bhatia and Malik 1991; Dewaraja and Sasaki 1991) and mental health issues that commonly present with depressive or anxiety symptoms. Several factors are responsible for Dhat syndrome. Generally, the conditions have been found mainly among young males from lower socioeconomic class groups who are rural residents and married (Arafat and Ahmed 2017; Kar et al. 2021). Although there is very limited research on Dhat syndrome, it has been found that Dhat syndrome is a manifestation of depression and has some association with somatoform disorders (Kar et al. 2021). Some myths around Dhat syndrome are the habit of masturbation, addiction to pornography, having sexual relationships with an impassionate woman, high sexual drives and homosexuality associated with Dhat syndrome (Prakash et al. 2018).

R. Kabir (✉) · A. D. Parsa
School of Allied Health, Anglia Ruskin University, Essex, UK
e-mail: russell.kabir@aru.ac.uk

M. Sivasubramanian · S. B. Mizan
Department of Nursing and Public Health, University of Sunderland, Sunderland, UK

© The Author(s), under exclusive license to Springer Nature Singapore Pte Ltd. 2024

S. K. Kar et al. (eds.), *Dhat Syndrome*,
https://doi.org/10.1007/978-981-99-8870-9_13

This chapter aims to review the public health aspects of Dhat syndrome, the stigma attached to Dhat syndrome, and different preventive measures.

## 13.2 Stigma Taboos Related to Sexuality

Dhat syndrome is an example of culture-informed sex obsession that is prevalent in the communities of the Indian subcontinent. Lipsedge and Littlewood (1985) argued that culture bound syndromes (CBS) (APA 2023) such as Dhat syndrome appear to be the reactions that are intermittent and intense amongst the particular communities (e.g., Indian subcontinent- South Asia; India and Southeast Asia and is also widespread in Nepal, Sri Lanka, Bangladesh, and Pakistan) (Mumford 1996; Sumathipala et al. 2004; Deb and Balhara 2013).

According to the American Psychological Association, it is "a pattern of mental illness and abnormal behaviour that is unique to a specific ethnic or cultural population and does not conform to standard classifications of psychiatric disorders" (ISSM 2023). Patients present with multiple symptoms, including sexual dysfunction (erectile dysfunction, premature ejaculation, and low libido), which causes a feeling of embarrassment or remorse. These are mainly due to culturally sensitive issues and stigmatised in the selected communities (ISSM 2023). Dhat syndrome represents a culture-related sex obsession and dysfunction attributed to the stigmatised sexuality accompanied by the loss of semen in nocturnal emission urine or masturbation (Wig 1960).

In patients with Dhat syndrome, due to both a neurotic and a culture-related disorder initiated by anxiety with the passage of semen, it is seen as a "cultural concept of distress" (Kar and Sarkar 2015). Sexual myths are passed through generations (Prakash 2007). One of the sexuality-related myths rooted in the era of Hippocrates and Aristotle was the concept of semen and sperm secretion. According to this belief, semen is considered to be an essential part of the body (i.e. "soul substance") (Deb and Balhara 2013) formed from the most perfected component of food". Reported by the Andrew Tissot myth of "losing one ounce of sperm is more debilitating than losing 40 ounces of blood.", is a western statement similar to the Indian myth (Prakash 2007).

Another example of a sexuality-related myth seen in Western European cultures indicated that losing semen by masturbation can cause significant mental disorders. This promoted the religious ban on masturbation (Prakash 2007). Previous research such as (Wen and Wang 1980; Behere and Natraj 1984; Bhatia and Malik 1991) has suggested that Dhat syndrome symptoms were common in unmarried or newly married young patients who were mainly from rural residents families with conservative views on sexuality (Deb and Balhara 2013). A study by Malhotra and Wig (1975) suggested that individuals from social class I had no taboo about sex and were less likely to worry about semen loss, whereas, in class IV, sex appeared as taboo. Patients diagnosed with Dhat syndrome thought the composition of Dhat was semen, pus, sugar, urine and even infection caused by masturbation and excessive pleasure in sexual activities, which has been associated with venereal diseases and UTI (Behere and Natraj 1984; Bhatia and Malik 1991). Although most literature has introduced Dhat syndrome as a male issue, some other evidence suggested the existence of a similar condition in females as "Dhat syndrome of females" predominantly presented with vaginal discharge (Kar and Sarkar 2015).

## 13.3 Myths and Misconceptions

Under a specific cultural setting-induced belief that sexual activity excessiveness causes Dhat disorder, it sounds reasonable when patients think their Dhat was because of reading erotic literature or pictures, watching pornographic movies, having unfulfilled desires, having lousy company, premarital or extramarital affairs, homosexuality, increased frequency of heterosexual sex (Jadhav 2004), unfaithfulness in love, sex during menstruation (Sumathipala et al. 2004; Bagadia et al. 1972; Gautham et al. 2008).

There have been other misconceptions, such as penile blood loss as a result of ejaculating semen (Prakash and Meena 2008) or semen flow out of the body causes loss of the "vital elixir of life" (Malhotra and Wig 1975). Though the views observing the preciousness of semen are limited to the Hindu religion's culture, there are somehow similar cultural values exist among followers of religions like Islam, Christianity, and Buddhism (Deb and Balhara 2013; Prakash et al. 2014; Sumathipala et al. 2004).

Another common myth amongst the Indian subcontinent places semen at the top of the hierarchy of bodily substances. This myth explains that 40 drops of food over 40 days converted into one drop of blood, where 40 drops of blood would form one drop of bone marrow, and finally and 40 drops of bone marrow be turned into one drop of semen (Prakash 2007; Prakash et al. 2014). Fear of semen loss has been disseminated widely through advertisements everywhere on walls, on television, in newspapers and on the roadside in many northern cities in India, leading to the patients' misconceptions. Therefore, they are getting lost in seeking proper medical services through psychiatrists rather than sexually transmitted diseased (STD) clinics, urologists and physicians (Prakash 2007).

## 13.4 Unawareness

Malhotra and Wig (1975) examined the link between Dhat syndrome and social class-related patients' knowledge of associated issues. Awareness about the normal sexual process was the least amongst patients from the social class IV. Another aspect of awareness is related to the availability of the correct information. Insufficient open communication within the family, particularly between parents and children, leaves young's awareness of the Dhat syndrome-related issues limited to a source of knowledge from their peers, who are equally less informed about the subject, leading to widespread misconceptions.

## 13.5 Public Health Impact of Dhat Syndrome

A study conducted in North India reported that most patients who suffer from Dhat syndrome prefer to consult with traditional healers and health specialists practising Ayurveda or Homeopathy and physicians before consulting with mental health professionals (Grover et al. 2016). The study further added that ayurvedic doctors are preferred most among all the indigenous practitioners for the patients in North India who suffer from Dhat syndrome. In their systematic review, Kar et al. (2021) identified that patients with Dhat syndrome take considerable time to seek treatment for Dhat syndrome. There is a delay of around 1.85 years before any treatment is sought. Singh et al. (2016) reported that for the first consultation, most of the patients went to unqualified practitioners (49.1%). It also has been reported that patients with Dhat syndrome do not regularly show up for follow-up visits. The probable reasons are that patients misunderstand that they are not suffering from any loss of semen and due to quick recovery (Chadda and Ahuja 1990). Grover et al. (2016), in their six monthly follow-up study with patients with Dhat syndrome reported that 45.3% of the patients had no change, 32.8% reported improved condition and 21.9% recovered from their symptoms. They also added that treatment completion was highly correlated with higher visits. Generally, the patients were self-referred to the first care provider and in 12.7% of cases, family members pushed them to seek healthcare advice (Singh et al. 2016). Shahi et al. (2022), in their cross-sectional investigation of a tertiary centre in North India, revealed that most of the patients were referred to them various departments of that tertiary centre and were presented with multiple sexual and psychiatric comorbidities. Menéndez et al. (2013) reported similar findings for a group of patients who went for a consultation with urologists in Spain, and the patients could end up with costly and unnecessary tests due to a lack of knowledge. Shahi et al. (2022) found that the quality of life and disability among patients with Dhat Syndrome compared to healthy individuals are poor.

## 13.6 Prevention of Dhat Syndrome

Generally, most people who suffer from "Dhat syndrome" do not first seek out professional care. Due to a lack of knowledge about existing health facilities and accompanying stigma, they consult with unlicensed medical professionals and elsewhere. Herbal remedies, dietary changes, protein-rich foods, antibiotics, B-complex pills or injections, advice from Vaids and Hakims, marriage can cure the symptoms, medications for anxiety, and sexual stimulants were taken by the Dhat syndrome patients; however, there is no evidence to support those that could be supported by science (Deb and Balhara 2013; Prakash et al. 2016). Also, it is frequently reported that those with Dhat syndrome are primarily given only medication, with their emotional and mental requirements being neglected. Medication can provide a short-term remedy for reducing the symptoms of depression, anxiety, and panic patients report experiencing. However, the actual source of the issue, their attitudes about semen, is unaffected. The primary symptoms of Dhat syndrome frequently improve with psychological treatments such as sex education, psychoeducation, counselling, and cognitive behaviour therapy (CBT) together with antidepressant and antianxiety drugs (Salam et al. 2012; Deb and Balhara 2013; Prakash et al. 2014; Kar and Sarkar 2015). In 2012, a cognitive behavioural therapy course that covered cognitive restructuring, sex education, imaginal desensitisation, relaxation training, and masturbatory training was created (Salam et al. 2012). For patients with Dhat Syndrome, CBT treatments are appropriate and effective (Tripathi and Sridevi 2014). Together with treatment, the prevention of Dhat syndrome needs serious attention. Dhat syndrome appears to be linked to poor sex education and sexual dysfunctions (Santos et al. 2017). According to systematic literature analysis, the average age of individuals with Dhat syndrome was 26 years (Udina et al. 2013). Public education and awareness should be conducted among young adults to control the health issues that result from Dhat syndrome (Sahu et al. 2015). To prevent Dhat syndrome following steps can be adopted, also shown in Fig. 13.1.

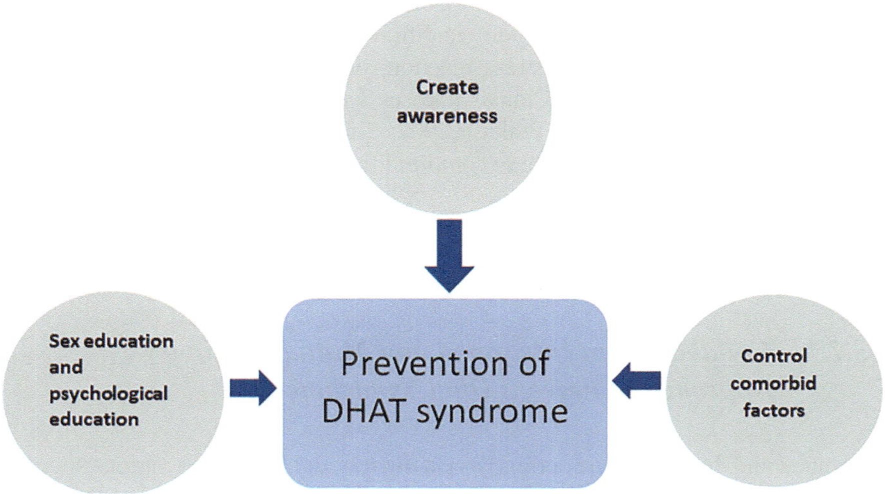


**Fig. 13.1** Prevention of Dhat syndrome

### 13.6.1 Create Awareness about Dhat Syndrome

Many people think that food gradually transforms into blood, marrow, and eventually semen. Some think cavernosal blood is expelled as semen after ejaculation (Deb and Balhara 2013; Prakash et al. 2016). So, creating awareness about Dhat syndrome is essential. Most Dhat syndrome patients learn about the condition from friends, family, coworkers, billboards, lay periodicals, and Vaids and Hakims (Deb and Balhara 2013; Prakash et al. 2016; Prakash 2007). Creating awareness and Education about Dhat syndrome is essential to prevent this syndrome.

### 13.6.2 Sex Education and Psychological Education

Dhat syndrome has been related to financial issues, bad company, seeing pornographic content, reading sexual stories, engaging in unhealthy habits like drunkenness, having unmet needs or desires, and being betrayed by friends or partners (Sumathipala et al. 2004; Gautham et al. 2008). To prevent Dhat syndrome focusing on these areas is needed. Proper sex education from the family and educational institutions can play a vital role.

### 13.6.3 Control Comorbid Factors

Dhat syndrome shares symptoms with several psychiatric conditions. Such as anxiety neurosis, depressive neurosis, hypochondriacal disorders, erectile dysfunction, premature ejaculation, and impotence (Dhikav et al. 2008; Prakash 2007; Singh 1985). The most prevalent comorbidity in different studies was depressive neurosis. Depressive psychosis, phobia, stress reaction, obsessive thinking, indications of physical dysmorphia, and delusional illnesses were among the other conditions identified (Dhikav et al. 2008; Prakash 2007; Singh 1985). To prevent Dhat syndrome, it is essential to control these comorbidities.

## 13.7 Other Public Health Perspectives

### 13.7.1 Collaboration, Integrated and Multidisciplinary Approach to Prevent Dhat Syndrome

Patients with Dhat syndrome currently visit doctors and learn from various sources. A combined strategy would benefit a more coordinated action to prevent Dhat syndrome. Dhat syndrome patients require a comprehensive preventive strategy, which a team approach could offer. Five main features of an integrated strategy for preventing Dhat syndrome can be considered (Fig. 13.2).

### *13.7.2 Collaboration Between Psychologists, Psychiatrists, and Psychological Social Workers*

A team effort and collaboration between psychiatrists and psychologists is essential to prevent and treat Dhat syndrome (Kar and Sarkar 2015). When people reach psychiatrists with anxiety, depression, and other psychological problems which may act as a comorbid factor for Dhat syndrome, they can provide sex education by referring those patients to a psychologist. Collaboration with social workers and providing training to social workers also can play a vital role. If trained and skilled, they can visit door-to-door to make people aware of Dhat syndrome and provide sex education. Media and newspapers also can broadcast awareness information related to Dhat syndrome.

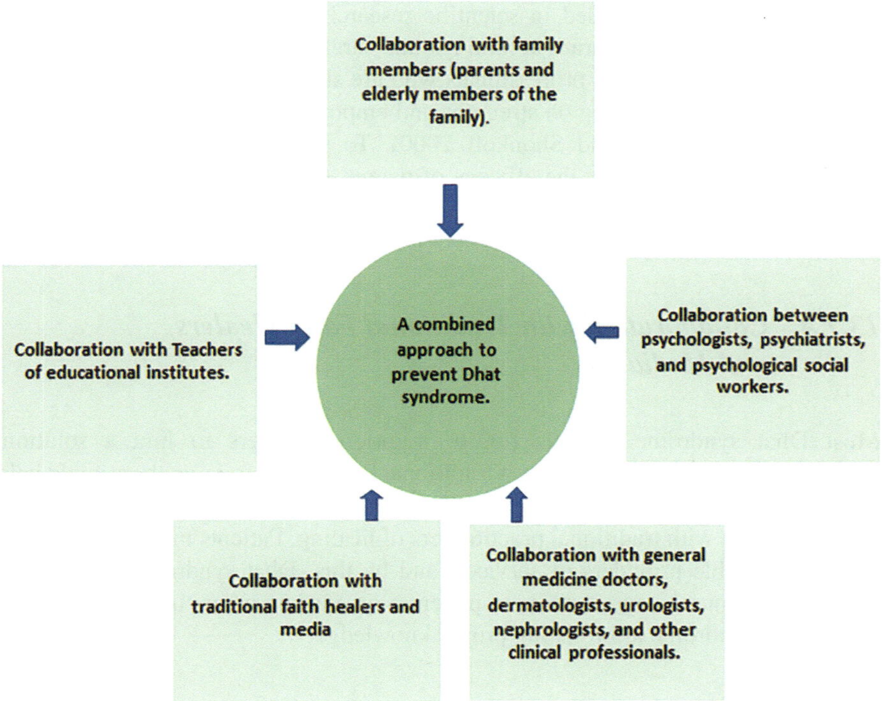


**Fig. 13.2** Combined strategy for preventing Dhat syndrome

### 13.7.3 Collaboration with Family Members

Individual-centred care is an all-encompassing management strategy emphasising the individual's unique characteristics in their environment. A broad model of care for Dhat syndrome may not adequately address the unique needs of each patient with a particular condition if it is attempted (Kar and Singh 2016). Families are therefore thought to be primarily responsible for ensuring that their children receive adequate sex education, acting as primary educational agents to prevent Dhat syndrome. Family members can play a vital role here. According to studies, parents often require support in the form of knowledge, inspiration, and tactics that might help them achieve the best results, even though they usually take on the responsibility of teaching their children about sexuality voluntarily (Vidourek et al. 2009; Bersamin et al. 2008; Goldman 2008). Sex education programmes for parents and legal guardians should be considered. Parenting programmes are events geared towards legal guardians and/or kids to enhance or modify the protective or vulnerability/risk elements that could affect a child's health and development (or overall well-being). According to Haberland and Rogow (2015), the research on parental programmes and sexuality education has, up until now, been viewed solely from a social, educational approach perspective and has strongly emphasised disseminating knowledge and fostering and enhancing communication.

Parenting programmes must possess a variety of characteristics, including a theoretical foundation grounded in scientific research, effortless availability, ethnic adequacy, adaptability, duration, timing, and strength, a community-based and family-centred orientation, professionals who are skilled and trained, personalised service delivery; developing on strengths and empowerment of families (Prinz and Sanders 2007; Phillips and Shonkoff 2000). To prevent Dhat syndrome, more research is needed to know the efficacy of parent- or family-centred interventions and programmes.

### 13.7.4 Collaboration with Traditional Faith Healers and Media

Most Dhat syndrome patients run to traditional healers to find a solution. Collaboration with the community's traditional healers and training them could help dispel the sexual stereotypes they pass on to the locals. The obstacle may be broken by cooperation with traditional practitioners of healing. Patients may be directed to the most suitable providers of services, and by this, Dhat syndrome can be prevented at the initial stage. And these patients can educate others in the community about Dhat syndrome after getting proper knowledge.

### *13.7.5 Collaboration with Multiple Medical Disciplines*

To this date, most individuals seeking treatment for Dhat syndrome go to general physicians and experts in alternative medicine rather than seeing a psychiatrist. Before seeing a psychiatrist (if at all), people with Dhat syndrome frequently seek out numerous additional consultations and obtain various information regarding sexual health, some of which may be at odds with one another. It can lead them astray and prevent them from receiving the proper care. The absence of Dhat syndrome from the curriculum for medical professionals trained in the Western system of medicine leaves them with inadequate awareness of the symptoms and treatment of this condition related to culture. An integrated approach would aim to deal with such individuals jointly and better educate the medical community about this illness. Integrating with multiple disciplines (general medicine doctors, dermatologists, urologists, nephrologists, and other clinical professionals) will provide a complete, more concentrated, socially and culturally acceptable form of care. Additionally, it will contribute to spreading uniform knowledge about sexual wellness and lowering the stigma linked to Dhat syndrome.

### *13.7.6 Collaboration with Teachers of Educational Institutes*

To prevent Dhat syndrome, collaboration with educational institutions is essential. However, early adolescence is the time when physiological processes like nocturnal emission start, so discussing natural sexual growth, anatomy of the genital system, and physiology of the genital system can help to prevent the development of Dhat syndrome; it might be beneficial to include sex education within the regular study curriculum. Teachers play a significant role in the success of school-based education programmes. According to studies, the capacity to educate is impacted by the teachers' dedication to and comfort with imparting sex education (Future of Sex Education Initiative). Teacher training on sex education is to increase teachers' commitment to the programme, increase their knowledge, and develop their abilities to deliver it. They should also emphasise the importance of programme integrity (LaChausse et al. 2014).

### *13.7.7 Sex Education Policy*

Sex education is defined as "an age-appropriate, culturally relevant approach to teaching about sex and relationships by providing scientifically accurate, realistic, non-judgmental information" (UNESCO). This concept indicates that sex education's goals go beyond simply imparting information on human anatomy, physiology of humans, reproduction, or STI prevention. Sex education, on the other hand, is approached integrally to educate young people about their sexual identities and relationships, eventually improving teenagers' reproductive health and general quality of life (WHO). Information regarding sexual and reproductive health is typically the focus of sex education. However, there are regional differences in sex education delivery methods, messaging, and content(Ramakoloi 2008). It is crucial to incorporate sex education from several sources to avoid Dhat syndrome. Programmes for sexual education may be offered in the community, at the family level, or in schools under the direction of educators, social workers, physicians, or other healthcare professionals. Sex education can be approached in many ways, including abstinence, abstinence-only, abstinence-only-until-marriage, and comprehensive sex education approaches.

### 13.7.8 Abstinence-Only-Until-Marriage or Abstinence-Only Education Approach

The Abstinence-only education (AOE) or abstinence-only-until-marriage (AOUM) programmes have religious roots and encourage total abstinence from all extramarital sex, even masturbation. Abstinence is seen from a philosophical perspective, emphasising the ideals of virginity and purity, and "teaches that a mutually faithful monogamous relationship in the context of marriage is the expected standard of human sexual behaviour." (Ehrlich 2006). The morals and character of students are crucial considerations. According to this strategy, rules prevent or restrict the inclusion of contraceptives in sex education, and skewed research frequently portrays contraceptive options (such as condoms and oral contraceptive pills) as ineffective. Advocates contend that educating students about contraception availability and use undermines the abstinence-only message and promotes immoral and health-harming sexual behaviours, raising the incidence of STDs and unintended pregnancies (Kirby 2001). However, conservative and religious organisations often support this strategy.

### 13.7.9 Abstinence Approach

While the Abstinence-only education and Abstinence-only until marriage approach view abstinence through an ethical lens, advocates of the abstinence approach view it as a behavioural and public health issue that encompasses actions like postponing sex, not having genital sex, and refusing to have additional sexual contact even after having had sexual experience. However, other sex-related activities, including hugging, kissing, joint masturbation, and anal and oral intercourse, are excluded from the definition of abstinence (Kohler et al. 2008).

### *13.7.10 Comprehensive Sex Education*

Abstinence is also covered in the curriculum for comprehensive sex education. However, Abstinence does not require promotion compared to the other methods. Instead, comprehensive sex education focuses on the value of safe sexual conduct and combines a variety of prevention measures for contraception to prevent STDs and unplanned pregnancies (Kohler et al. 2008). The protection of human rights, gender parity, participatory learning, youth activism, civic participation, and cultural sensitivity are ideals and practices that are ingrained in comprehensive sex education, which is an empowerment-based field. It seeks to give students the information, perspectives, and abilities they need to make decisions that will advance their sexual health (Haberland and Rogow 2015; Boonmongkon and Thaweesit 2009). For instance, contrary to popular belief and a report from the United Nations Population Fund (2022), comprehensive sex education does not result in early sexual initiation or risky sexual behaviour.

Teenagers and young adults frequently lack the resources necessary to find reliable information regarding sexual issues, which increases their concerns about such subjects. They are prone to receiving inaccurate information from informal sources. A lack of appropriate sexual education will negatively impact adolescent growth. Giving them the right pieces of information from suitable sources could ease their worries and stop the fear of semen loss from arising.

## 13.8 Conclusion

There are a lot of myths about Dhat syndrome among the general people. The majority of people think that losing sperm while urinating will make them infertile or in some other way sexually inferior. This cultural mentality contributes to the fact that Dhat syndrome is frequently accompanied by feelings of shame, worry, and despair. It is crucial that people who suffer from Dhat syndrome should seek immediate support and need to improve their sexual health education. Health education that involves sexual health education would improve awareness amongst the most vulnerable group (i.e. young adults) in those particular conservative societies (e.g. South Asia). This could include the anatomy and physiology of sex organs and the simplified explanation of function (e.g. semen, nocturnal emissions and masturbation). Public health interventions, including health promotion strategies and health education at the broader community level and, in particular, integrated with formal education at the school level, which targets teenagers and college students, would remove misconceptions and raise the awareness that finally impacts psychological and physical health.

## References


American Psychological Association (APA). Dictionary of Psychology—"Culture-bound syndrome". 2023. Available at: https://dictionary.apa.org/culture-bound-syndrome. Accessed 6 June 2023.

Arafat SM, Ahmed S. Burden of misconception in sexual health care setting: a cross-sectional investigation among the patients attending a psychiatric sex clinic of Bangladesh. Psychiatry J. 2017; https://doi.org/10.1155/2017/9827083.

Avasthi A, Nehra R. Sexual disorders: a review of Indian research. In: Murthy RS, editor. Mental health in India (1995–2000). Bangalore: People's Action for Mental Health; 2001. p. 42–53. https://doi.org/10.4103/psychiatry.IndianJPsychiatry_716_20.

Bagadia V, Dave K, Pradhan P, Shah L. A study of 258 male patients with sexual problems. Indian J Psychiatry. 1972;14:143–51.

Behere PB, Natraj GS. Dhat syndrome: the phenomenology of a culture-bound sex neurosis of the orient. Indian J Psychiatry. 1984;26:76–8.

Bersamin M, Todd M, Fisher DA, Hill DL, Grube JW, Walker S. Parenting practices and adolescent sexual behavior: a longitudinal study. J Marriage Fam. 2008;70(1):97–112. https://doi.org/10.1111/j.1741-3737.2007.00464.x.

Bhatia MS, Malik SC. Dhat syndrome—a useful diagnostic entity in Indian culture. Br J Psychiatry. 1991;159:691–5.

Boonmongkon P, Thaweesit S. Sexuality education in Thailand: how far do we need to go. ARROWS for Change. 2009;15(2/3):12–3.

Chadda RK, Ahuja N. Dhat syndrome: a sex neurosis of the Indian subcontinent. Br J Psychiatry. 1990;156(4):577–9.

De Silva P, Dissanayake SA. The use of semen syndrome in Sri Lanka: a clinical study. Sex Marital Ther. 1989;4:195–204.

Deb KS, Balhara YPS. Dhat syndrome: a review of the world literature. Indian J Psychol Med. 2013;35(4):326–31. https://doi.org/10.4103/0253-7176.122219.

Dewaraja R, Sasaki Y. Semen loss syndrome: a comparison between Sri Lanka and Japan. Am J Psychother. 1991;45:14–20.

Dhikav V, Aggarwal N, Gupta S, Jadhavi R, Singh K. Depression in Dhat syndrome. J Sex Med. 2008;5(4):841–4. https://doi.org/10.1111/j.1743-6109.2007.00481.x.

Ehrlich JS. From age of consent laws to the silver ring thing: the regulation of adolescent female sexuality. Health Matrix. 2006;16:151.

Gautham M, Singh R, Weiss H, Brugha R, Patel V, Desai NG, Grosskurth H. Socio-cultural, psychosexual and biomedical factors associated with genital symptoms experienced by men in rural India. Tropical Med Int Health. 2008;13(3):384–95. https://doi.org/10.1111/j.1365-3156.2008.02013.x.

Goldman JD. Responding to parental objections to school sexuality education: a selection of 12 objections. Sex Educ. 2008;8(4):415–38. https://doi.org/10.1080/14681810802433952.

Grover S, Avasthi A, Gupta S, Dan A, Neogi R, Behere PB, Lakdawala B, Tripathi A, Chakraborty K, Sinha V, Bhatia MS. Phenomenology and beliefs of patients with Dhat syndrome: a nationwide multicentric study. Int J Soc Psychiatry. 2016;62(1):57–66. https://doi.org/10.1177/0020764015591857.

Haberland N, Rogow D. Sexuality education: emerging trends in evidence and practice. J Adolesc Health. 2015;56(1):S15–21. https://doi.org/10.1016/j.jadohealth.2014.08.013.

International Society for Sexual Medicine (ISSM). (2023). What is dhat syndrome?, Available at https://www.issm.info/sexual-health-qa/what-is-dhat-syndrome. Accessed 6 June 2023.

Jadhav S. Dhat syndrome: a re-evaluation. Psychiatry. 2004;3:14–6.

Kar SK, Menon V, Arafat SY, Singh A, Das A, Shankar A, Sharma P, Perera S. Dhat syndrome: systematic review of epidemiology, nosology, clinical features, and management strategies. Asian J Psychiatr. 2021;65:102863. https://doi.org/10.1016/j.ajp.2021.102863.

Kar SK, Sarkar S. Dhat syndrome: evolution of concept, current understanding, and need of an integrated approach. J Hum Reprod Sci. 2015;8(3):130. https://doi.org/10.4103/0974-1208.165143.
Kar SK, Singh A. Person centered management approach for the Dhat syndrome. Int J Pers Cent Med. 2016;6:4. https://doi.org/10.5750/ijpcm.v6i4.615.
Kirby D. Emerging answers: research findings on programs to reduce teen pregnancy (summary). Am J Health Educ. 2001;32(6):348–55. https://doi.org/10.1080/19325037.2001.10603497.
Kohler PK, Manhart LE, Lafferty WE. Abstinence-only and comprehensive sex education and the initiation of sexual activity and teen pregnancy. J Adolesc Health. 2008;42(4):344–51. https://doi.org/10.1016/j.jadohealth.2007.08.026.
LaChausse RG, Clark KR, Chapple S. Beyond teacher training: the critical role of professional development in maintaining curriculum fidelity. J Adolesc Health. 2014;54(3):S53–8. https://doi.org/10.1016/j.jadohealth.2013.12.029.
Lipsedge M, Littlewood R. Transcultural psychiatry. In: Granville-Grosman, editor. Recent advances in clinical psychiatry. 3rd ed. Edinburgh: Churchill Livingstone; 1985.
Malhotra HK, Wig NN. Dhat syndrome: a culture-bound sex neurosis of the orient. Arch Sex Behav. 1975;4:519–28.
Menéndez V, Fernández-Suárez A, Placer J, García-Linares M, Tarragon S, Liso E. Dhat syndrome, an emergent condition within urology in Spain. World J Urol. 2013;31:941–5. https://doi.org/10.1007/s00345-012-0911-4.
Mumford DB. The "Dhat syndrome": a culturally determined symptom of depression? Acta Psychiatr Scand. 1996;94:163.
Phillips DA, Shonkoff JP, (eds.). From neurons to neighborhoods: the science of early childhood development. National Academies Press (US). National Research Council (US) and Institute of Medicine (US) Committee on Integrating the Science of Early Childhood Development 2000. https://doi.org/10.17226/9824.
Prakash O. Lessons for postgraduate trainees about Dhat syndrome. Indian J Psychiatry. 2007;49(3):208. https://doi.org/10.4103/0019-5545.37324.
Prakash O, Kar SK. Dhat syndrome: a review and update. J Psychosexual Health. 2019;1(3–4):241–5. https://doi.org/10.1177/2631831819894769.
Prakash O, Kar SK, Rao TS. Indian story on semen loss and related Dhat syndrome. Indian J Psychiatry. 2014;56(4):377. https://doi.org/10.4103/0019-5545.146532.
Prakash O, Meena K. Association between Dhat and loss of energy: a possible psychopathology and psychotherapy. Med Hypotheses. 2008;70:898–9. https://doi.org/10.1016/j.mehy.2007.09.010.
Prakash S, Sharan P, Sood M. A study on phenomenology of Dhat syndrome in men in a general medical setting. Indian J Psychiatry. 2016;58(2):129. https://doi.org/10.4103/0019-5545.183776.
Prakash S, Sharan P, Sood M. A qualitative study on psychopathology of dhat syndrome in men: implications for classification of disorders. Asian J Psychiatr. 2018;35:79–88. https://doi.org/10.1016/j.ajp.2018.05.007.
Prinz RJ, Sanders MR. Adopting a population-level approach to parenting and family support interventions. Clin Psychol Rev. 2007;27(6):739–49. https://doi.org/10.1016/j.cpr.2007.01.005.
Ramakoloi BK. Sexuality education in Sweden-a study based on research and young people's service providers in Gothenburg. Gothenburg, Sweden: Gothenburg University; 2008. https://gupea.ub.gu.se/bitstream/handle/2077/17923/gupea_2077_17923_1.pdf?sequence=1&isAllowed=y. Accessed 26 May 2013
Sahu RN, Sharma VK, Kumar A, Bavishi C, More B. Dhat syndrome and its association with sexual behavior and pyschiatric comorbidities in males: a case control study. Int J Med Res Health Sci. 2015;4(1):90–3. https://doi.org/10.5958/2319-5886.2015.00015.6.
Salam KA, Sharma MP, Prakash O. Development of cognitive-behavioral therapy intervention for patients with Dhat syndrome. Indian J Psychiatry. 2012;54(4):367. https://doi.org/10.4103/0019-5545.104826.
Santos M, Rocío RN, Valdes M. In: Sharpless BA, editor. Unusual and rare psychological disorders: a handbook for clinical practice and research. Oxford University Press; 2017. https://doi.org/10.1093/med:psych/9780190245863.003.0016. (2016). Accessed 10 May 2023.

Shahi MK, Tripathi A, Singh A, Kar SK, Nischal A, Singh S, Dalal PK. Quality of life and disability in patients with Dhat syndrome: a cross-sectional study. Indian J Psychol Med. 2022;44(5):459–65. https://doi.org/10.1177/02537176221078422.

Singh A, Tripathi A, Gupta B, Agarwal V. Pathways to care for dhat (semen loss anxiety) syndrome: a study from North India. Int J Ment Health. 2016;45(4):253–61. https://doi.org/10.1080/00207411.2016.1238741.

Singh G. Dhat syndrome revisited. Indian J Psychiatry. 1985;27(2):119–22.

Sumathipala A, Siribaddana SH, Bhugra D. Culture-bound syndromes: the story of dhat syndrome. Br J Psychiatry. 2004;184(3):200–9. https://doi.org/10.1192/bjp.184.3.200.

Tripathi M, Sridevi G. CBT in Dhat syndrome and co-morbid conditions. Int J Sci Res Publ. 2014;4(9):1–8.

Udina M, Foulon H, Valdés M, Bhattacharyya S, Martín-Santos R. Dhat syndrome: a systematic review. Psychosomatics. 2013;54(3):212–8. https://doi.org/10.1016/j.psym.2012.09.003.

United Nations Population Fund.(2022). Comprehensive sexuality education. Available online: https://www.unfpa.org/comprehensive-sexuality-education. Accessed 25 May 2023.

Vidourek RA, Bernard AL, King KA. Effective parent connectedness components in sexuality education interventions for African American youth: a review of the literature. Am J Sex Educ. 2009;4(3–4):225–47. https://doi.org/10.1080/15546120903408974.

Wen JK, Wang CL. Shen-kui syndrome: a culture-specific sexual neurosis in Taiwan. In: Kleinman A, Lin TY, editors. Normal and abnormal behaviour in Chinese culture. Dordrecht, Holland: D Reidel Publishing Co; 1980. p. 357–69.

Wig NN. Problems of mental health in India. J Clin Soc Psychiatry. 1960;17:48–53.

# Chapter 14
# Current Research and Gaps in Dhat Syndrome

**Nishtha Laspal and Siddharth Sarkar**

## 14.1 Introduction

Dhat syndrome is sexual neurosis commonly found in the South Asian population. Classically, it is described as an overwhelming concern about semen loss through urine or nocturnal emissions, leading to a perceived loss of vitality and consequent weakness of the body. It is a clinical consideration not only in India but cases of Dhat syndrome have been reported in other countries as well, primarily among males of South Asian ethnicity. According to a systematic review of Dhat syndrome, it is commonly diagnosed in the South Asian population (Kar et al. 2021b). Much of the scientific literature on Dhat syndrome is focused on phenomenology and some other aspects like management or outcomes are less frequently discussed.

For any psychiatric condition to be understood thoroughly, comprehensive, contextual and continued research is important to gather knowledge about the disorder. Research directions about psychiatric disorders may have many facets, including understanding the presentation and phenomenology, the aetiology and theoretical underpinnings in bio-psycho-social terms, the clinical assessment and management of patients, lived experiences and outcomes, policy and therapeutic perspectives, and many more. This chapter is not a comprehensive evaluation of all the research on Dhat syndrome but provides a snapshot of some relevant research (primarily of the last 10 years), key research gaps, few methodological considerations, and potential future research directions. Some aspects of ongoing research may also be covered in the other chapters of the book.

N. Laspal · S. Sarkar (✉)
Department of Psychiatry and National Drug Dependence Treatment Centre, All India Institute of Medical Sciences, New Delhi, India

© The Author(s), under exclusive license to Springer Nature Singapore Pte Ltd. 2024

S. K. Kar et al. (eds.), *Dhat Syndrome*,
https://doi.org/10.1007/978-981-99-8870-9_14

## 14.2 Current Research Directions on Dhat Syndrome

A lot of research has accrued in the field of Dhat syndrome, reflected by bibliometric findings (Kar et al. 2021a). By 2021, there were 89 articles on Dhat syndrome on Scopus. Most of the literature on this topic, according to this bibliometric analysis has come from the Postgraduate Institute of Medical Education and Research (PGIMER), Chandigarh; All India Institute of Medical Sciences (AIIMS), New Delhi; and King George's Medical University (KGMU) Lucknow. The current research directions are discussed further under phenomenology, risk factors and aetiology, comorbidities (primarily psychiatric), assessment and scales, and interventions.

### *14.2.1 Phenomenology*

There have been numerous attempts to understand the multi-dimensional aspects of Dhat syndrome (schematically shown in Fig. 14.1). Dhat syndrome is widely understood as a culture-bound syndrome, though some authors disagree. Studies on the phenomenology of Dhat syndrome have described it as culture-reactive syndrome, idioms of distress and sex neurosis. Some deem it not to be culture-specific at all. Traditional studies view Dhat syndrome as a physical disorder rather than a

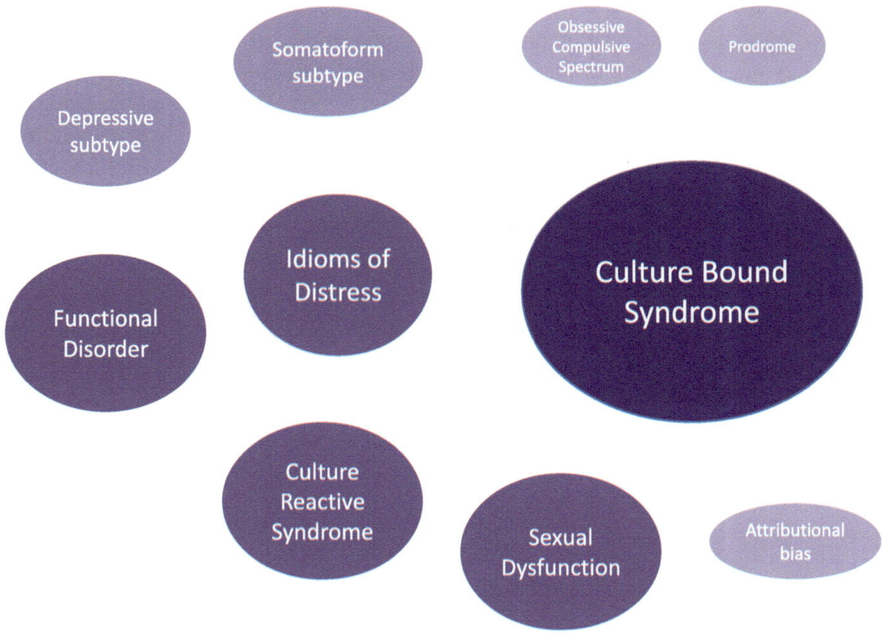


**Fig. 14.1** Schematic representation of phenomenological aspects of Dhat syndrome

psychological one. Many attempts have been made in the last decade to gain a better understanding of Dhat syndrome, but its correct understanding continues to elude researchers to date.

In a study conducted on 100 adult males attending a community sex and marriage clinic in India, the phenomenology of Dhat syndrome was studied (Prakash et al. 2016). The majority of patients were young adult males in the 20 to 30-year age group, unmarried and reported passage of Dhat through urine. Most of them also had associated depressive, anxiety, and somatic symptoms during presentation. Loss of masculinity, erectile dysfunction and premature ejaculation were the most common sexual symptoms reported. The study found that majority had mild to moderate symptoms and associated mild distress and dysfunction in cases of Dhat syndrome. The authors conceptualized Dhat syndrome to be closer to an internalizing disorder rather than an externalizing one. They also identified three clusters—I (mild symptoms), II (most severe symptoms), and III (moderate symptoms) based on the severity of symptoms. They found younger age and more co-morbidity associated with severe symptomatology.

A case from India reported the phenomenon of neutralization behaviour in a man with Dhat syndrome where the man drank his semen after masturbation to preserve the 'vital force' or Dhat from his body (Agrawal et al. 2022). A morbid case about a man who presented with a history of chronic self-mutilation of his penis owing to distress from his perceived loss of semen through urine required a penile reconstruction surgery (Maheshwari et al. 2022). This case highlights the serious risks involved in selected untreated cases of Dhat syndrome.

Although there have been numerous cases of semen loss from other body parts, an unusual case from Bangladesh reported about a man who believed that rotten semen was being collected in his mouth and excreted in his saliva (Arafat et al. 2022). Another unusual presentation of loss of Dhat was reported through the anus (Balhara and Goel 2012). In a rare case of Dhat syndrome by proxy, a young boy was brought by his father who attributed the loss of semen from his son during nocturnal emissions to his son's poor growth (Hafi et al. 2022), and sought medicines to cut down his son's desire and nocturnal emissions for his son to grow well.

An unusual case of Koro and Dhat syndrome co-morbid with an obsessive-compulsive disorder in a young male was reported by authors and they suggested screening for obsessive-compulsive spectrum in all cases of culture-bound syndromes (Ghosh and Chowdhury 2020). A case from India described Dhat syndrome during the prodrome of schizophrenia, broadening the varied symptom domains found during the prodromal phase (Kar et al. 2017). A study done in 2016 hypothesized the development of sexual dysfunction followed by the attribution of cause to the cultural concept of Dhat (Rajkumar 2016). This attribution leads to further worsening of sexual functions and reinforcement of Dhat syndrome.

Anthropological research on the Dhat syndrome as idioms of distress is an area of growing interest and may provide a better understanding of its socio-cultural aspects and provide an acceptable way to study without the stigma of psychiatric illness. It may help in better therapeutic engagement and consequently fewer drop-outs from treatment (Kaiser and Jo Weaver 2019).

A few case reports of Dhat syndrome from several countries have also been published in the last decade, challenging the notion that Dhat syndrome is limited to the Indian subcontinent. A novel case of Dhat syndrome was reported in a native male from Oman, who presented with typical clinical features (Uvais 2017). Similar to India, the patient had contact with traditional healers first before seeking mental health services. Previous studies have shown cases of Dhat syndrome in Spain, Japan, Sri Lanka, and Russia although many of these cases included emigrants from the Indian subcontinent (Kar and Sarkar 2015). Western literature on Dhat syndrome usually involves case reports of emigrants from South Asia who present to clinics with a similar presentation of somatic complaints without any apparent medical illness and attribution of cause to semen loss or sometimes sugar loss in the urine (Ilzarbe et al. 2021). Encountering such a clinical presentation becomes challenging for Western physicians who often miss the cultural context of these populations and patients are sometimes misdiagnosed and unsatisfied with treatment. Western literature has acknowledged time and again that culture-bound syndromes are often overlooked when addressing people of different ethnicities (Kim et al. 2020).

There has been a growing interest in female Dhat syndrome in the last decade, however, studies are still scarce. In a study done in India, 70 women with non-pathological vaginal discharge were assessed and found to experience multiple vague bodily symptoms and attributed them to vaginal discharge similar to Dhat syndrome in males (Joshi et al. 2022). The majority of these females reported stressful situations before the onset of illness. In yet another study of 69 females with non-pathological discharge, similar attribution of the loss of vaginal fluid with loss of 'vital' fluid from the body and experiencing multiple physical symptoms was observed (Mehra et al. 2021). The study of Dhat syndrome in females remains an under-researched area compared to males.

### *14.2.2 Treatment Pathways*

According to a nationwide multicentric study involving 780 patients with Dhat syndrome, the mean duration of illness was found to be 4.26 years (a standard deviation of 4.4 years) before their first contact with health services. The mean age of presentation was 23.9 years (standard deviation of 8.5 years) (Grover et al. 2016a). This was in keeping with most of the previous studies done on Dhat syndrome.

Another Indian study of pathways to care for Dhat Syndrome found a marked delay in presenting to a medical professional with a mean of 6.78 years (standard deviation 6.94) (Grover et al. 2016c). In this study, Ayurveda, Yoga, Unani, Siddha and Homoeopathy (AYUSH) practitioners were found to be the first choice by patients.

In a 6-month follow-up study of 64 patients with Dhat syndrome, 64% of patients dropped out of treatment citing "no improvement with treatment", "not prescribed medications" and logistic issues (Grover et al. 2016b). Treatment outcome at the end of 6 months showed treatment completers perceived improvement but only 34% reported satisfaction with treatment. Treatment completers were found to have better knowledge and understanding of sex and had sought treatment themselves compared to the dropout subjects.

### 14.2.3 Risk Factors

Studies on Dhat syndrome found male gender, young age of onset, lower education levels, low socio-economic status and rural background to be most commonly seen in Dhat syndrome (Grover et al. 2016c). However, there is literature to suggest higher education levels and urban backgrounds in patients with Dhat Syndrome (Singh et al. 2021). Conservative knowledge and attitude regarding sexual practices, being unmarried and Hindu religion were found to be more common in Dhat syndrome (Prakash et al. 2016).

A study on patients with Dhat syndrome found high performance anxiety, substance dependence and childhood adversities as significant risk factors for developing Dhat syndrome later in life (Rajkumar 2016). A study conducted to investigate any common genetic link between Dhat syndrome and depression found patients with a positive family history of depression had higher rates of co-morbid depressive disorders and substance use disorder than patients without any family history. This finding might support the notion that Dhat syndrome may be a variant of the depressive spectrum (Rajkumar and Bharadwaj 2014).

### 14.2.4 Comorbidity and Disability

Dhat syndrome is often seen with psychiatric as well as medical co-morbidities. Some estimate that around one-third of patients with Dhat syndrome may be suffering from co-morbid psychiatric illness. Among patients with Dhat syndrome, major depression, anxiety and substance use disorder were more prevalent (Prakash et al. 2016). Overall most studies found depression followed by anxiety and somatization disorder in patients with Dhat syndrome (Strong et al. 2022). Sexual dysfunction has also been reported, where a majority of individuals with Dhat syndrome suffer from premature ejaculation followed by erectile dysfunction and loss of libido (Grover et al. 2015). Some of the common medical comorbidities are urinary tract infections and sexually transmitted diseases.

A cross-sectional study done in India found poor quality of life and disability amongst patients with Dhat syndrome (Shahi et al. 2022). Those patients while those who had medical or psychiatric co-morbid conditions had a poorer quality of life and higher disability compared to those without any co-morbidities.

### 14.2.5 Measurement and Assessment of Dhat Syndrome

Diagnostic instruments for Dhat syndrome are few and the majority have been developed in the last decade. A study conducted in a community clinic in India came up with an operational definition of Dhat syndrome based on information collected from various stakeholders such as patients, psychiatrists, other medical specialists and alternative medicine practitioners (Prakash et al. 2016). They also developed a diagnostic tool for Dhat syndrome using focused group discussions and items from a previous scale by the authors (Dhat syndrome interview schedule). They came up with an 18-item Dhat disorder diagnostic interview and a 47-item Dhat disorder severity scale which included health beliefs and associated symptoms of somatic, anxiety, depressive, cognitive and sexual symptoms.

Dhat syndrome questionnaire (DSQ) was developed for the evaluation of Dhat syndrome by Grover et al. (2014). The DSQ is an 18-item, self-rated questionnaire and was found to have good content validity and is available in both Hindi and English. The authors further modified the DSQ to assess the female equivalent of Dhat syndrome and developed the Scale for Assessment of Female Dhat syndrome questionnaire (SAFeD) (Grover and Shouan 2020).

### 14.2.6 Interventions

Some of the major challenges in treating Dhat syndrome include a lack of awareness in the community, delay in treatment-seeking and lack of management options. In a follow-up study, Grover studied treatment challenges faced while managing Dhat syndrome patients. The main factors for dropout included poor sexual knowledge and negative attitude towards sexuality (Grover et al. 2016b).

Studies on interventions for Dhat syndrome are relatively few. A study done in NIMHANS in 2012 was the first of its kind to develop a cognitive behavioural therapy module for Dhat syndrome. This included basic sex education, cognitive restructuring, imaginal desensitization, Kegel's exercise, relaxation and other techniques such as masturbation homework, and imaginal desensitization (Salam et al. 2012). The study reported improvement in symptoms; however, the module was applied to only five patients and had no comparison group. An article from 2015 proposed an integrated approach to manage Dhat syndrome which included mental health professionals, other medical professionals and traditional, complementary and alternative medicine practitioners to help bridge the treatment gap (Kar and Sarkar 2015).

The Clinical Practice Guidelines for the assessment of sexual dysfunction by the Indian Psychiatric Society in 2017 advised taking a history of Dhat syndrome in all patients with sexual dysfunction and the use of the Dhat Syndrome Questionnaire in suspected cases (Avasthi et al. 2017). It also advised the treatment of Dhat syndrome before the management of erectile dysfunction or premature ejaculation. It also formulated a treatment algorithm for patients with Dhat syndrome which included exploring co-morbid psychiatric, medical illness or sexual dysfunction and treatment where necessary. Management with basic knowledge of sex and clarifications of misconceptions regarding it were advised. Prakash et al. (2016) proposed sex education, psychotherapy including cognitive behaviour therapy & brief solution-focused therapy along with psychoeducation, relaxation techniques and medications if needed, such as anxiolytics and antidepressants for comprehensive management. Some clinicians have given trials of anti-psychotics with good responses in patients with Dhat syndrome (Ilzarbe et al. 2021). A two-session therapy was proposed, targeted especially for non-psychiatrists to help them manage patients of Dhat syndrome in the community (Innamuri and Ramaswamy 2021). The author elucidates a stepwise approach to these patients in two visits requiring 30–45 minutes each session.

### *14.2.7 Methodological Issues in Dhat Syndrome Research*

Based on the current state of evidence, there are certain methodological issues and challenges identified in the research about Dhat syndrome. The first challenge pertains to the definition of Dhat syndrome per se. Many researchers have reported on the variants of Dhat syndrome. There is a need to have an evolved consistent definition of Dhat syndrome. A lack of common consensus regarding its phenomenology, nosology and management further impedes research in this area of study.

The second methodological challenge pertains to Dhat syndrome being a hidden population, often away from conventional medical care. Individuals with Dhat syndrome are reluctant to discuss this in the family or a busy outpatient clinic, and often present with vague somatic symptoms and some forms of 'weakness'. Thus, getting adequate samples which are reflective of the community sample may be elusive.

The third methodological issue pertains to the lived experience of individuals with Dhat syndrome. Western medicine and traditional Indian systems of medicine do not converge on the necessity of conserving semen. What is pathologized in one system of medicine is not necessarily so in another. Conflicting information about 'Dhat' may lead to reporting biases or treatment retention/engagement of the individuals with Dhat syndrome.

## 14.3 Research Gaps and Way Forward

Some research gaps could be identified based on the present evaluation of the current state of research on Dhat syndrome (Table 14.1). Most studies are observational and there is a dearth of interventional studies in Dhat syndrome. Exploration of different treatment approaches can help to find out which treatment works and for which kind of patients.

**Table 14.1** Research gaps and the way forward for Dhat syndrome

| Research gap | Way forward |
| --- | --- |
| Lack of interventional studies | Development and efficacy evaluation of intervention modules or evaluation of pharmacotherapies for Dhat syndrome |
| The longitudinal course of illness is not clearly established | Longitudinal cohort studies, ascertaining fluctuations and impact of marriage/ sexual partnership |
| Biological research limited | Exploratory studies to understand the biological correlates of the disorder. |
| Understanding the economic impact of Dhat syndrome limited | Cost of illness studies (including direct costs, indirect costs and treatment costs) |
| The burden of Dhat syndrome and its impact scarcely studied | Quality of life and disease burden can be assessed systematically |
| Lack of community-based studies | Community-based studies designed to tap hidden populations, ensuring some kind of privacy |
| Impact of sex education as a preventive measure | A trial design (ecological, quasi-experimental or randomized) to see whether sex education can result in reduced rates of genesis of Dhat syndrome. |
| Research in women, individuals who identify as LGBTQIA | Further targeted research in these populations |
| Definition of Dhat syndrome | Consensus operational definition of Dhat syndrome for research and clinical purposes through a consultative epistemological framework |

There are very scarce studies investigating the longitudinal course of Dhat syndrome patients and the natural course of this illness is still unknown. Thus, there is a need to understand the longitudinal course of Dhat syndrome, ascertain fluctuations, and know whether marriage or sexual partnership leads to amelioration of Dhat syndrome.

Several studies on Dhat syndrome are exploring the sociocultural aspects of Dhat syndrome. However, no studies have been done to understand its biological basis. Exploratory research into biological aspects of Dhat syndrome can be helpful (for example, attentional biases towards sexual themes, reactance towards health and bodily physiological symptoms, etc.).

Many studies have shown that patients with Dhat syndrome suffer from long-standing illness and disability, and undergo numerous consultations and investigations before reaching mental health services. Despite this knowledge, there has been no cost of illness studies done on Dhat syndrome, which can help us better to understand the economic impact of Dhat syndrome on patients and families.

Quality of life, the burden of disease (and caregiver burden or distress) are also rarely studied for Dhat syndrome. If the findings are significant, this can help drive further research by involving multiple stakeholders.

Almost all of the studies are hospital-based samples and there is a lack of community-based studies. Community-based studies can be useful. Snowball sampling is unlikely to work for Dhat syndrome, and other methods of data sample recruitment (for example, anonymous telephone contact, advertisements through small notices in public transport, and contacting alternate healthcare providers) may be useful.

Even though the research on Dhat syndrome itself is scarce, studies on females are relatively lesser and to our knowledge no study on Dhat syndrome in LGBTQ individuals. Research may explore whether LGBTQIA individuals also experience Dhat syndrome (where both qualitative and quantitative approaches may be useful).

Whether sex education can work as a preventive measure for Dhat syndrome has not yet been studied. One could consider an ecological, quasi-experimental or randomized study by delivering sex education in higher classes in schools and assessing the subsequent rates of development of Dhat syndrome.

Literature to date has not been able to come up with a unitary definition of Dhat syndrome. The phenomenology of Dhat syndrome continues to be a matter of debate. The nosological status of Dhat syndrome also continues to be elusive since culture-bound syndromes are difficult to categorize in existing conventional categories of Western classificatory systems. Efforts should be made to codify the operational and clinical definition of Dhat syndrome.

## 14.4 Conclusion

Dhat syndrome is recognized as a culture-bound syndrome, prevalent in the Indian sub-continent. Recent studies have been studying its phenomenology, nosology and management. However, the majority of the research related to Dhat syndrome has been done to understand the phenomenology of Dhat syndrome. There is a need to expand research horizons through concerted, collaborative and astute research endeavours.

## References

Agrawal AK, Bagewadi V, Das S, Moirangthem S. Recycling of semen: a rare phenomenon in Dhat syndrome. Psychiatr Danub. 2022;34(2):313–4. https://doi.org/10.24869/psyd.2022.313.

Arafat SMY, Mondal F, Ghimire S. A 47-year-old man passing putrid semen through saliva and sweat: a case of Dhat syndrome. J Gen Fam Med. 2022;23(3):177–9. https://doi.org/10.1002/jgf2.513.

Avasthi A, Grover S, Sathyanarayana Rao T. Clinical practice guidelines for Management of Sexual Dysfunction. Indian J Psychiatry. 2017;59(5):91. https://doi.org/10.4103/0019-5545.196977.

Balhara YPS, Goel R. An unusual presentation of Dhat syndrome. J Neuropsychiatry Clin Neurosci. 2012;24(3):E19–20. https://doi.org/10.1176/appi.neuropsych.11070153.

Ghosh S, Chowdhury AN. A case of two culture-bound syndromes (Koro and Dhat syndrome) coexisting with obsessive–compulsive disorder. Indian J Psychiatry. 2020;62(2):221–2. https://doi.org/10.4103/psychiatry.IndianJPsychiatry_298_19.

Grover S, Avasthi A, Aneja J, Shankar G, Mohan M, Nehra R, Padhy SK. Comprehensive questionnaire for assessment of Dhat syndrome: development and use in patient population. J Sex Med. 2014;11(10):2485–95. https://doi.org/10.1111/jsm.12241.

Grover S, Avasthi A, Gupta S, Dan A, Neogi R, Behere PB, Lakdawala B, Tripathi A, Chakraborty K, Sinha V, Bhatia MS, Patjoshi A, Rao TSS, Rozatkar A. Phenomenology and beliefs of patients with Dhat syndrome: a nationwide multicentric study. Int J Soc Psychiatry. 2016a;62(1):57–66. https://doi.org/10.1177/0020764015591857.

Grover S, Gupta S, Avasthi A. Psychological correlates and psychiatric morbidity in patients with Dhat syndrome. Indian J Psychiatry. 2015;57(3):255–61. https://doi.org/10.4103/0019-5545.166637.

Grover S, Gupta S, Avasthi A. A follow-up study of patients with Dhat syndrome: treatment pattern, outcome, and reasons for dropout from treatment. Indian J Psychiatry. 2016b;58(1):49. https://doi.org/10.4103/0019-5545.174373.

Grover S, Gupta S, Mahajan S, Avasthi A. Pathway of care among patients with Dhat syndrome attending a psychosexual clinic in tertiary care center in North India. Ind Psychiatry J. 2016c;25(1):72–7. https://doi.org/10.4103/0972-6748.196040.

Grover S, Shouan A. Assessment scales for sexual disorders—a review. J Psychosexual Health. 2020;2(2):121–38. https://doi.org/10.1177/2631831820919581.

Hafi B, Uvais NA, Varughese A, Aysha S. Dhat syndrome by proxy: an underreported entity. Prim Care Companion CNS Disord. 2022;24(2):21cr02993. https://doi.org/10.4088/PCC.21cr02993.

Ilzarbe L, Ilzarbe D, Arbelo N, Llach C, Anmella G, Vieta E, Murru A. Dhat syndrome: a case report on a culture-bound challenge. Eur Psychiatry. 2021;64(Suppl 1):S733. https://doi.org/10.1192/j.eurpsy.2021.1941.

Innamuri R, Ramaswamy D. Demystifying Dhat syndrome: a two-session therapy proposal. J Psychosexual Health. 2021;3(3):270–4. https://doi.org/10.1177/26318318211023876.

Joshi S, Tripathi A, Agarwal S, Singh N, Gupta B, Nischal A, Kar SK. Phenomenology, disability and sexual functioning in female Dhat syndrome: a study of tertiary care gynaecology outpatients. Gen Psychiatr. 2022;35(5):e100863. https://doi.org/10.1136/gpsych-2022-100863.

Kaiser BN, Jo Weaver L. Culture-bound syndromes, idioms of distress, and cultural concepts of distress: new directions for an old concept in psychological anthropology. Transcult Psychiatry. 2019;56(4):589–98. https://doi.org/10.1177/1363461519862708.

Kar SK, Arafat SY, Menon V. A bibliometric analysis of Dhat syndrome. Psychiatr Int. 2021a;2(4):379–85.

Kar SK, Menon V, Arafat SY, Singh A, Das A, Shankar A, Sharma P, Perera S. Dhat syndrome: systematic review of epidemiology, nosology, clinical features, and management strategies. Asian J Psychiatr. 2021b;65:102863. https://doi.org/10.1016/j.ajp.2021.102863.

Kar SK, Sarkar S. Dhat syndrome: evolution of concept, current understanding, and need of an integrated approach. J Hum Reprod Sci. 2015;8(3):130–4. https://doi.org/10.4103/0974-1208.165143.

Kar SK, Shahi MK, Tripathi A. Dhat syndrome as the prodrome of schizophrenia: understanding the cultural distress. Asian J Psychiatr. 2017;25:203–4. https://doi.org/10.1016/j.ajp.2016.11.006.

Kim G, Wang SY, Park S, Yun SW. Mental Health of Asian American older adults: contemporary issues and future directions. Innov Aging. 2020;4(5):igaa037. https://doi.org/10.1093/geroni/igaa037.

Maheshwari PN, Tillu ND, Shah US. Extreme self-mutilation due to "Dhat" syndrome. Indian J Urol. 2022;38(3):243–4. https://doi.org/10.4103/iju.iju_94_22.

Mehra A, Kathirvel S, Gainder S, Avasthi A, Grover S. Female Dhat syndrome in primary care setting. Ind Psychiatry J. 2021;30(2):278–84. https://doi.org/10.4103/ipj.ipj_76_20.

Prakash S, Sharan P, Sood M. A study on phenomenology of Dhat syndrome in men in a general medical setting. Indian J Psychiatry. 2016;58(2):129–41. https://doi.org/10.4103/0019-5545.183776.

Rajkumar RP. Distinctive clinical features of Dhat syndrome with comorbid sexual dysfunction. Asian J Psychiatr. 2016;19:1–2. https://doi.org/10.1016/j.ajp.2015.11.004.

Rajkumar RP, Bharadwaj B. Dhat syndrome: evidence for a depressive spectrum subtype. Asian J Psychiatr. 2014;9:57–60. https://doi.org/10.1016/j.ajp.2014.01.007.

Salam KPA, Sharma MP, Prakash O. Development of cognitive-behavioral therapy intervention for patients with Dhat syndrome. Indian J Psychiatry. 2012;54(4):367–74. https://doi.org/10.4103/0019-5545.104826.

Shahi MK, Tripathi A, Singh A, Kar SK, Nischal A, Singh S, Dalal PK. Quality of life and disability in patients with Dhat syndrome: a cross-sectional study. Indian J Psychol Med. 2022;44(5):459–65. https://doi.org/10.1177/02537176221078422.

Singh A, Karthik MS, Viswanathan S, Sathianathan AR. Dhat syndrome—revisiting the phenomenology and related psychiatric comorbidities. J Psychosexual Health. 2021;3(1):73–7. https://doi.org/10.1177/2631831820979301.

Strong YN, Li A, White ME, Razzak AN, Anderson DJ, Kaye AD, Herron EW, Khater NP, Bradley EC, Urits I. Dhat syndrome: epidemiology, risk factors, comorbidities, diagnosis, treatment, and management. Health Psychol Res. 2022;10(4):38759. https://doi.org/10.52965/001c.38759.

Uvais NA. Dhat syndrome among the Islamic populations of India and Pakistan. Oman Med J. 2017;32(5):442. https://doi.org/10.5001/omj.2017.84.

# Chapter 15
# Dhat Syndrome: A Fact or Myth

**Mohammad Muntasir Maruf, Tamkeen Saleem, and S. M. Yasir Arafat**

## 15.1 Introduction

Culture affects almost every aspect of our life at least in some forms. It evolves over time and influences the thoughts and behaviour of individuals (Lehman et al. 2004). Some specific syndromes exist in some cultures. A culture-bound syndrome is a pattern of mental illness that is unique to a specific ethnic or cultural population and these patterns do not conform to the standard classifications of psychiatric disorders (American Psychiatric Association 2013). These patterns are indigenously reflected as illnesses and mostly have local names. The physical and mental health classification systems like the *International Classification of Diseases (ICD-10)*, and the *Diagnostic and Statistical Manual of Mental Disorders* fifth edition (DSM-5) give comprehensive and structured information regarding the cultural viewpoints that can facilitate the assessment of psychiatric illnesses.

Dhat syndrome is a culture-bound syndrome prevalent mostly in South Asia. It is a diagnostic category that frames a comprehensible understanding of specific recurring, preset and distressing experiences that mimic the phenomenology of neurotic spectrum disorders (Prakash and Kar 2019). It is typified by a clinical picture including preoccupation and undue concern about excessive semen loss through ejaculation, nocturnal emission, urine, or other means (Strong et al. 2022; Avasthi and Jhirwal 2005). The existence of the belief that there are debilitating effects of semen loss on health and that semen preservation is constructive to the physical and

M. M. Maruf
Department of Addiction Psychiatry, National Institute of Mental Health, Dhaka, Bangladesh

T. Saleem
Department of Clinical Psychology, Shifa Tameer-e-Millat University, Islamabad, Pakistan

S. M. Y. Arafat (✉)
Department of Psychiatry, Enam Medical College and Hospital, Dhaka, Bangladesh

© The Author(s), under exclusive license to Springer Nature Singapore Pte Ltd. 2024

S. K. Kar et al. (eds.), *Dhat Syndrome*,
https://doi.org/10.1007/978-981-99-8870-9_15

psychological health of a man is a conception mutually shared in the community (Khan 2005).

## 15.2 Evolving of Dhat Syndrome

Semen has been considered a "soul substance" for a long. The work by *Galen* and *Aristotle* revealed a strong linkage of physiological and mental well-being with its loss. In Indian traditions, "Virya" i.e. semen signifies vigor and it is perceived as a basis for the physical and spiritual vitality of men. Therefore, the perception prevails that the loss of virya via any erotic act or imagination for example masturbation or *swapnadosh* i.e. wet dreams is harmful to physical and spiritual health (Nag 1996; Verma et al. 2003). However, the issue of *dhat* or belief that semen loss weakens the body and causes the disease is not restricted to Hindus only, rather it is widespread among all communities of South Asian cultures. The prevalence of dhat has been registered in other South Asian groups like Sikhs in India, Buddhists in Sri Lanka and Muslims in Pakistan (as *mardana kamzori)* (Mumford 1996). *Mardana kamzori* is a generic term that is characterized as inability to maintain erection, and ejaculation, engendered by local myths of thinning of semen, masturbation and wet dreams (Khan 2005). Dhat syndrome predominantly prevails in young and single men mostly having rural backgrounds and low levels of education (Chadda and Ahuja 1990; Grover et al. 2015; Kar and Sarkar 2015; Khan 2005; Singh 1985). The mean age of onset of symptoms is 19 years of age (Dhikav et al. 2008). Dhat syndrome patients exhibit illness behaviours such as hypochondriasis and emotional distress. It is manifested in the form of anxiety and somatic complaints like weakness, dizziness, sleep problems, fatigue, backache, and leanness. It is alleged to be connected with losing semen through masturbation, immoderate intercourse, nocturnal emission or urine (Bottéro 1991; Wen and Wang 1981). South Asian females also tend to account for a similar set of manifestations attributing the symptomology to vaginal discharge (Patel et al. 2005). Females who may report dhat syndrome, their symptoms are attributed to vaginal discharge and are diagnosed as other psychiatric disorders like somatoform, mood and anxiety disorders (Kar and Singh 2017).

## 15.3 Myths and Help-Seeking

Based on enduring beliefs and lack of proper sexual health literacy, loss of semen provides a plausible and acceptable explanation for the symptoms and distress the persons suffer. Such beliefs help them to express their need for help and to be accepted by others from the same cultural background. Promotion of the need for treatment for such conditions by traditional healers encourages to seek help from persons who support the beliefs (Balhara 2011). Consistent with the prevailing myths, studies have shown that close friends, relatives, local traditional healers, quacks, or advertisements by *Ayurvedic* practitioners are considered as the source of information about the importance of semen for most patients (Prakash 2007). Men from rural India seek help for their sexual problems including dhat syndrome mostly from traditional practitioners who follow the systems of *Ayurveda*, *Unani*, *Siddha*, *Homeopathy* etc. In the cases where patients ultimately reach the mental health professional or psychiatrist, they do it late, after following a long pathway of care and visiting various other practitioners (Grover et al. 2016a). According to a study from North India, before consulting a mental health professional, patients delay around 6.8 years (Grover et al. 2016b). Another study reported that patients with Dhat syndrome sought help for the first time after a mean duration of about 1.8 years, and from that point, they consulted a mental health professional after around 4.6 years (Singh et al. 2016). Moreover, there is a high dropout rate from treatment, probably due to the patient's dissatisfaction with the explanation of the syndrome they are offered. Self-referred patients are more likely to complete the treatment than patients who are referred by other professionals (Grover et al. 2016c).

## 15.4 Myths in Dhat Syndrome

### *15.4.1 Myths Related to Phenomenology*

#### 15.4.1.1 Myth: Semen Is a Source of Vitality

The term 'Dhat syndrome' was introduced in the scientific literature first by N. N. Wig, a psychiatrist in India (Wig 1960). The word *Dhat* has been derived from the word "Dhatu", is a Sanskrit (a classical language belonging to the Indo-Aryan subdivision of the Indo-European languages) word; English meaning of which is "Metal" or "Elixir". In the context of the disorder, the second meaning, i.e., "Elixir" is emphasized here. The myths surrounding the syndrome are originally related to the essence of "Dhatu". The knowledge and beliefs regarding "Dhatu" prevailed from the system, culture and documents dated thousand years back (Prakash et al. 2014).

Ayurveda, the ancient Indian alternative medicine system, based on a pseudoscientific natural and holistic approach to human health described the importance of seven "Dhatus" or essential components of the body. According to the Ayurveda, human health is all about the balance between seven dhatus - *Rasa* (Chyle), *Rakta* (Blood), *Mamsa* (Flesh), *Meda* (Fat), *Asthi* (Bone), *Majja* (Marrow) and *Shukra* (Semen), "Shukra Dhatu" aka "Veerya" being the most important one—the force of life (Thakar 2010).

According to the *Charaka Samhita,* a Sanskrit text on Ayurveda, semen is prevailing within the body like "oil in the sesame seed" and the optimal yearly ejaculation for humans is 168 times. The *Shiva Samhita,* a Sanskrit text on yoga, mentioned semen as a seed and emphasized that a man should hold his seed with all his power because the falling of the seed leads to death. Ayurveda says that excessive ejaculation or frequent intercourses results in wastage of semen (according to *Charaka Samhita - Sukra Kshya*) resulting in a decline in vigour and vitality and various diseases. "Kama Sutra" by Vatsayana (300 AD), the historical and famous Indian literature on sexual activities, also emphasizes the pivotal role of semen in maintaining the health of the individual (Grover et al. 2016c; Prakash et al. 2014; Deb and Balhara 2013).

Ayurvedic documents resonate with the belief of Hinduism regarding semen. Other religious cultures including Islam, Buddhism and Christianity also emphasize the importance of the preservation of semen mentioning the harmful effects of semen loss on the body and mind (Kar and Sarkar 2015). According to a group of Islamic scholars, ejaculation of semen by masturbation is forbidden and considered a shameful offence or sin in their religion. Some Buddhist monks retain their semen to have a long energetic life as they believe that, the whole body contains semen which is the source of energy derived from the refinement of food (Prakash et al. 2014).

Not only in ancient Indian regions but in various cultures and in various periods throughout the world, semen got a highly precious mention. According to *Hippocrates* (460–377 BC), semen provides the form of the human body. *Galen* (130–201) compared losing sperm to losing vital spirits. Andrew Tissot (1728–97) echoed Indian literature by opining that losing one ounce of sperm was more incapacitating than losing 40 ounces of blood (Sumathipala et al. 2004).

So, semen is a *Dhatu* of so overwhelming importance that too many become ultimately semen. The belief prevails that losing semen causes an imbalance of "Dhatus" in our body, draining the body off all its energy that would have been derived from food, resulting in physical weakness and illness. Therefore, semen loss-related disorder has been mentioned as the "Dhat syndrome", where the loss of semen is equivalent to the loss or imbalance of all the 'Dhatus' (Rao 2021). But, some people perceive dhat broadly as any whitish discharge (Arafat 2017). Some authors describe the disorder as "semen loss-related psychological distress", "semen loss syndrome", "semen loss anxiety" etc. (Kar et al. 2021a, b; Prakash 2007).

#### 15.4.1.2 Fact: Semen Does Not Contain any Physical Energy

Semen is important in the process of reproduction. Semen enables the survival of spermatozoa and acts as a medium through which they reach the female reproductive system. Various components of semen lubricate the urethral opening and remove any urine residue from the urethra before ejaculation and ensure that sperm can better stay within the female reproductive tract (Mawhinney and Mariotti 2013). Fertility issues are indispensably related to sperm count and quality, but there is a lack of evidence to conclude that ejaculation frequency is related to general health outcomes. Moreover, masturbation is scientifically recognized as a common sexual behaviour among adults without any deleterious medical consequences (Mascherek et al. 2021).

#### 15.4.1.3 Myth: Semen Is Formed from Foods through Multistep Processes

Semen is believed to be formed through a multistep process of purification and filtration of foods. This belief originates from the Indian ancient literature, dated between the fifth millennium BC and the seventh century AD, which claims that one drop of blood is formed from 40 drops of food, one drop of the flesh is composed of 40 drops of blood, one drop of marrow is formed from 40 drops of flesh and 40 drops of marrow ultimately form one drop of semen and each step of this process of forming semen from food takes 40 days to be completed (Arafat 2017). Some others like Bramhacharya literature, claim this value to be 100 drops instead of 40 (Chakraborty et al. 2020). *Aristotle* (384–322 BC) also believed that sperms are the extract of as well as the most perfect component of our food (Prakash 2007). Some people believe that through ejaculation, the cavernosal blood is drained as semen (Prakash and Meena 2008).

#### 15.4.1.4 Fact: There Is no Direct Relationship Between Semen and Food

Semen is composed of the spermatozoa from the vas deferens and secretions of the seminal vesicles, prostate, and bulbourethral glands – the parts of the male reproductive system, the main bulk being the seminal vesicle fluid (almost 60% of the total volume of semen). During ejaculation, contractions of the smooth muscles of the epididymis propel the sperm into the vas deferens, which deliver the sperm to the ejaculatory duct by joining with the seminal vesicle duct near the prostate. The seminal vesicles release mucoid material, containing fructose, citric acid, and other nutrient substances, that amalgam with the sperm to form semen. In the ejaculatory duct, alkaline fluid from the prostate and thick fluid from the bulbourethral glands or Cowper's glands are added to the semen. The usual volume of semen per ejaculation is 1.5–5 ml which normally contains 39 million or more sperm. Usually, men produce millions of new sperm every day and a sperm regeneration cycle (spermatogenesis) *takes about 74 days on average (*Amann 2008*;* Mawhinney and Mariotti 2013; Mascherek et al. 2021).

### *15.4.2 Myths Related to Symptom Presentation*

#### 15.4.2.1 Myth: Dhat Syndrome Is a Disorder of Males from a Rural Background

Dhat syndrome is regarded as a disorder in males. Indian studies depicted the prototype of such patients as unmarried or recently married males with low socioeconomic status living in a rural background (Rao 2021).

#### 15.4.2.2 Fact: Females Also Suffer from Similar Symptoms

Irrespective of marital status, individuals from any residential background can be affected by the syndrome (Mawhinney and Mariotti 2013). A Bangladeshi study showed that more than half the participants with complaints of semen loss were married and more than three-fourths were from an urban background (Maruf et al. 2021). Another study from Bangladesh also revealed that misconceptions were not associated with educational attainment (Arafat and Ahmed 2017). Recently, some authors claimed of finding a similar syndromal pattern in some females who presented with the symptoms of whitish vaginal discharge associated with physical and psychological symptoms as seen in dhat syndrome among males. Therefore, they suggested the existence of "Female Dhat Syndrome" (Chaturvedi 1988; Grover et al. 2014a, b).

#### 15.4.2.3 Myth: Semen Is Wasted through Masturbation, Night Emission and Urine

Many people believe that ejaculation through other than sexual intercourse results in loss of semen which in turn leads to dilution of semen concentration that causes other physical and psychological consequences (Kar et al. 2021a, b). Whitish discharge mixed with urine or after urination is regarded as semen loss by many (Deb and Balhara 2013). Pre-ejaculatory clear fluid is also considered semen by many (Arafat 2017). In an Indian study, more than one-third of the respondents believed that night emissions more than once a week were abnormal (Verma et al. 2003). In a study conducted on Bangladeshi males, around three-fourths of them believed that involuntary emission of semen while sleeping, which they termed *swapnadosh*, occurred due to sexual diseases and sexual weakness (Miah et al. 2015). One report identified that the patient believed that semen is lost through sweat and saliva (Arafat et al. 2021).

#### 15.4.2.4 Fact: Masturbation Is a Normal Physiological Process

Though it is discouraged by religions, masturbation, according to medical science, is a natural way of dealing with sexual urges, for which no ill effects have been found. Negative effects of masturbation are caused by feelings of "masturbatory guilt" (the guilt felt by the individuals who masturbate but at the same time despise it as morally disgraceful) and not by the behaviour itself (Aneja et al. 2015). Rather some studies reported that masturbation exhibits an abundance of positive effects on both mental and physical health (Herbenick et al. 2023). Whitish discharge through urine may be caused by various conditions including phosphaturia, chyluria, proteinuria, pyuria etc. (Saha et al. 2012). Pre-ejaculatory fluid, primarily produced from bulbourethral glands, is chemically different from semen, and it comes out of normal sexual arousal to act as a lubricant and acid neutralizer (Chudnovsky and

Niederberger 2007). Night emission is a part of the normal sexual developmental process which is most common during adolescence and early adulthood though it can happen any time after puberty.

#### 15.4.2.5 Myth: Semen Loss Causes Physical and Mental Illness

Patients with Dhat syndrome assume the loss of semen causes irreversible damage to the body resulting in various physical symptoms and illnesses including neurasthenia, fatigue, anaemia, leprosy, and tuberculosis (Rao 2021). George Beard (1838–1883) claimed that the depletion of sexual energy, often through nocturnal or involuntary emissions is one of the commonest reasons for neurasthenia (Prakash 2007). Sigmund Freud (1856–1939) believed that the source of neurasthenia is masturbation and the frequency of it is proportional to male neurasthenia (Sumathipala et al. 2004). Several Indian studies reported that most people believe that besides sexual problems loss of semen causes non-sexual symptoms, too (Rao 2021). Henry Maudsley (1835–1918) regarded that loss of semen, mainly through masturbation, results in severe mental illness (Sumathipala et al. 2004). A Bangladeshi study reported that about 92% of participants believed that masturbation causes mental illness (Miah et al. 2015).

#### 15.4.2.6 Fact: There Is no Evidence-Based Explanation for Semen Loss and Physical and Mental Illness

There is no evidence of a biological association between ejaculation through nocturnal emissions or masturbation and the above-mentioned conditions (Whorton 2001). In the last century, neurasthenia as a diagnosis eventually came to be seen as a mental and behavioural rather than a physical condition. But it is no longer included in DSM by *American Psychiatric Association* and is deprecated in the latest version of the ICD-11 (Connor 2022). Self-reported mental problems may be considered as an expression of a discrepancy between moral beliefs and behaviour.

#### 15.4.2.7 Myth: Semen Loss Leads to Sexual Problems and Infertility

Patients with Dhat syndrome believe that semen loss will lead to the inability to procreate male descendants, early death of offspring, deformed fetus, permanent impotency, and deformed size and shape of the penis (Strong et al. 2022). A large multicentric study in India reported that more than three-fourths of the individuals with Dhat syndrome believe that semen loss leads to reduced sexual ability (Grover et al. 2016a). In another study, half of the respondents having sexual dysfunctions attributed the problem to semen loss (Chadda and Ahuja 1990).

#### 15.4.2.8 Fact: There Is no Proof of Infertility Due to Dhat Syndrome

Current evidence does not show any relationship of sexual dysfunction with semen loss (Rao 2021). Rather, myths regarding semen loss can affect an individual psychologically which can in turn hamper sexual performance. On the other hand, fertility issues are related to the quality of sperm and long abstinence does not guarantee improved quality (Hanson et al. 2018). Before semen collection for evaluation of the quality, World Health Organization recommended an ejaculatory abstinence period is 2–7 days to get improved semen parameters (World Health Organization (WHO) 2010). But the recommendation has been challenged as the evidence is inconclusive (Mascherek et al. 2021).

### *15.4.3 Myths Related to Treatment*

#### 15.4.3.1 Myth: Dhat Syndrome Can Be Treated by Changes in Diet and Sexual Behaviour

In an earlier study, people were found to believe that modifying dietary habits and avoiding masturbation, bad company and erotic literature, dhat syndrome can be cured. Marriage was also a solution believed by some (Malhotra and Wig 1975). In a recent study, dietary changes as well as taking energizing tablets and injections, taking medications to increase sexual desire and reduce infection, applying certain creams on genitals etc., were reported as a cure by the respondents (Grover et al. 2016a). Ayurveda mentions certain foods and behaviours which it claims to prevent semen loss (Thakar 2010).

#### 15.4.3.2 Fact: Changing the Belief Is Vital

Varied treatment strategies like dietary and herbal "supplements", protein and iron-rich diet, antibiotics, multivitamins etc., have been used but related scientific evidence is sparse (Deb and Balhara 2013; Arafat 2017). Sex education focusing on a basic understanding of anatomy, physiology, and functions of sexual organs concerning masturbation, semen formation, nocturnal emissions and clarifying sexual myths is important as treatment approaches (Kar and Sarkar 2015). Other psychotherapeutic measures like psycho-education, relaxation techniques, brief solution-focused therapy, cognitive behaviour therapy as well as medications like anti-depressants and anxiolytics in the least possible doses in case of co-morbid anxiety or/depression are recommended (Rao 2021). Patients need multifaceted intervention, which can be provided through a multidisciplinary team approach (involving psychiatrists, clinical psychologists, psychiatric nurses, and psychiatric social workers) supported by close liaison with the general physicians, dermatologists, venereologists, and alternative medicine practitioners (Kar and Sarkar 2015;

Udina et al. 2013). Some authors advocated for a person-centred management approach including empathic listening, non-confrontational attitude, individualized care and collaborative approaches as an effective model of care for such patients (Kar and Singh 2016).

## 15.5 Dealing with Myths

### *15.5.1 Sex Education*

There is no alternative to educating people to deal with dhat syndrome while combating the myths (Table 15.1). Sex education involving the basic understanding of normal sexual development and anatomy and physiology of the reproductive system may be integrated into the regular educational curriculum (Arafat 2017). Early adolescence is the period when physiological processes like nocturnal emission and responding to sexual arousal by masturbation start. But during that crucial period, adolescents do not have reliable sources for gaining appropriate information about sexual issues. Sex education explaining the sexual myths by family and teachers may help prevent the development of Dhat syndrome (Kar and Sarkar 2015; Kar et al. 2021a, b). Clinicians should delve into efforts to educate patients with dhat syndrome.

**Table 15.1** Commonly available myths and facts regarding Dhat syndrome

| Myths | Facts |
|---|---|
| Semen is a source of vitality | Semen does not contain any physical energy |
| Semen is formed from foods through multistep processes | There is no direct relationship between semen and food |
| Dhat syndrome is a disorder of males from a rural background | People from urban backgrounds and females also suffer from similar symptoms |
| Semen is wasted through masturbation, night emission and urine | – Masturbation is a normal physiological process<br>– Night emission is a part of normal development<br>– Whitish colour of urine has been attributed to various physiological and pathological reasons, not to semen |
| Semen loss causes physical and mental illness | There is no evidence-based explanation for semen loss and physical and mental illness |
| Semen loss leads to sexual problems and infertility | – There is no direct relationship between semen loss and sexual problems<br>– There is no proof of infertility due to Dhat syndrome |
| Dhat syndrome can be treated by changes in diet and sexual behaviour | – Changing the belief is vital<br>– Various psychosocial measures and in some cases, psychotropics are helpful |

### 15.5.2 Public Awareness Campaigns

Awareness programs regarding the myths through an organized process of communication targeting the lay public may be an effective approach. Like any other anti-stigma campaign, such awareness programs also should include policymakers, politicians, celebrities from media and sports etc.

### 15.5.3 Mass Media Campaigns

Mass media due to its tremendous reach and constant exposure can play vital roles in the prevention of unauthentic dissemination of myths and misconceptions regarding sexual health (Arafat 2017). Besides print and electronic media, nowadays social media has become a powerful platform to build and disseminate awareness as it is widely used and some platforms provide a relatively safer and welcoming atmosphere for people (Chen 2021).

### 15.5.4 Enhanced Research

Research should be patronized possibly by investing in scaling up research infrastructures and allocating research funds for collaborative research proposals (Kar and Singh 2016).

### 15.5.5 Multidisciplinary Collaboration

As dhat syndrome is managed by a variety of professionals ranging from traditional practitioners to psychiatrists, there should be a collaborative approach among all the concerned disciplines and an efficient referral system to demystify the disorder. In this context, a collaboration of psychiatrists with specialists from other disciplines including general medicine, dermatology and venereology, urology, sexual medicine practitioners, and neurology as well as with professionals from allied disciplines like psychology, clinical psychology, psychiatric nursing and psychiatric social work is important (Kar and Sarkar 2015). More important is the collaboration of the modern medical system with the alternative systems of medicine and Ayurvedic, Homeopathic, Unani, Siddha and alike traditional practitioners. The role of local religious and political leaders is also note-worthy. There should be more dialogue, discussion, information and knowledge sharing among all the stakeholders involved in the management of Dhat syndrome (Rao 2021; Arafat 2017). Besides ensuring culturally acceptable and effective treatment, such collaboration will help reducing stigma, imparting uniform information, breaking the barrier of appropriate referral and resolving the myths the traditional healers hold and disseminate (Arafat 2017).

### *15.5.6 Specialized Service Centers and Proper Referral*

Specialized services targeting sexual health problems could be established. Besides, a proper and effective referral system should be established starting from primary health care (Arafat and Ahmed 2017).

## 15.6 Conclusions

Various kinds of myths exist regarding dhat syndrome in the cultures of the Indian sub-continent like, dhat syndrome is a disorder of males from a rural background; semen is the source of vitality, which is formed from foods through multi-step processes; through urine, night emission and masturbation, semen is wasted which leads to physical, mental and sexual problems. Such myths affect the help-seeking behaviours of the patients who visit traditional healers and are mistreated by non-scientific management approaches. In this chapter, we highlighted the prevailing myths and explained the evidence-based facts. Various measures including multi-disciplinary collaboration among concerned professionals, the establishment of specialized service centres and a proper referral system, inclusion of sex education in the school curriculum, arranging public awareness programs, encouraging high-quality research and responsible contribution of media are warranted to deal with myths. We hope that knowledge about the existing myths regarding dhat syndrome and reliable scientific information against those will be helpful for the people in the prevention and management of the problem.

## References

Amann RP. The cycle of the seminiferous epithelium in humans: a need to revisit? Int J Androl. 2008;29(5):469–87. https://doi.org/10.2164/jandrol.107.004655.

American Psychiatric Association. Diagnostic and statistical manual of mental disorders. Washington, DC; 2013.

Aneja J, Grover S, Avasthi A, Mahajan S, Pokhrel P, Triveni D. Can masturbatory guilt lead to severe psychopathology: a case series. Indian J Psychol Med. 2015;37(1):81–6. https://doi.org/10.4103/0253-7176.150848.

Arafat SMY. Dhat syndrome: culture bound, separate entity, or removed. J Behav Health. 2017;6(3):147–50. https://doi.org/10.5455/jbh.20170123102726.

Arafat SMY, Ahmed S. Burden of misconception in sexual health care setting: a cross-sectional investigation among the patients attending a psychiatric sex Clinic of Bangladesh. Psychiatry J. 2017;2017:9827083. https://doi.org/10.1155/2017/9827083.

Arafat SMY, Mondal F, Ghimire S. A 47-year-old man passing putrid semen through saliva and sweat: a case of Dhat syndrome. J Gen Fam Med. 2021;23(3):177–9. https://doi.org/10.1002/jgf2.513.

Avasthi A, Jhirwal OP. The concept and epidemiology of Dhat syndrome. J Pak Psychiatr Soc. 2005;2(1):6–8.

Balhara YP. Culture-bound syndrome: has it found its right niche? Indian J Psychol Med. 2011;33(2):210–5. https://doi.org/10.4103/0253-7176.92055.

Bottéro A. Consumption by semen loss in India and elsewhere. Cult Med Psychiatry. 1991;15(3):303–20.

Chadda RK, Ahuja N. Dhat syndrome. A sex neurosis of the Indian subcontinent. Br J Psychiatry. 1990;156:577–9. https://doi.org/10.1192/bjp.156.4.577.

Chakraborty A, Mukhopadhyay D, Mandal AK, Ghosh S. Study of Dhat syndrome in men in West Bengal: a clinic-based study. J Psychosexual Health. 2020;2(3–4):260–4. https://doi.org/10.1177/2631831820939000.

Chaturvedi S. Psychasthenic syndrome related to leucorrhea in Indian women. J Psychosom Obstet Gynecol. 1988;8:67–72.

Chen X. The effect of media representations and stigma on public perception of mental disorders from late 20th to early 21st century. Adv Soc Sci Educ Humanit Res. 2021;615:622–5.

Chudnovsky A, Niederberger CS. Copious pre-ejaculation: small glands—major headaches. J Androl. 2007;28(3):374–5. https://doi.org/10.2164/jandrol.107.002576.

Connor H. Doctors and ‘educational overpressure’ in nineteenth-century Britain: a fatigue state that divided medical opinion. Eur J History Med Health. 2022;79:1–36. https://doi.org/10.1163/26667711-bja10026.

Deb KS, Balhara YP. Dhat syndrome: a review of the world literature. Indian J Psychol Med. 2013;35(4):326–31. https://doi.org/10.4103/0253-7176.122219.

Dhikav V, Aggarwal N, Gupta S, Jadhavi R, Singh K. Depression in Dhat syndrome. J Sex Med. 2008;5(4):841–4. https://doi.org/10.1111/j.1743-6109.2007.00481.x.

Grover S, Avasthi A, Aneja J, Shankar G, Mohan M, Nehra R, Padhy SK. Comprehensive questionnaire for assessment of Dhat syndrome: development and use in patient population. J Sex Med. 2014b;11(10):2485–95. https://doi.org/10.1111/jsm.12241.

Grover S, Avasthi A, Gupta S, Dan A, Neogi R, Behere PB, Lakdawala B, Tripathi A, Chakraborty K, Sinha V, Bhatia MS, Patjoshi A, Rao TS, Rozatkar A. Phenomenology and beliefs of patients with Dhat syndrome: a nationwide multicentric study. Int J Soc Psychiatry. 2016a;62(1):57–66. https://doi.org/10.1177/0020764015591857.

Grover S, Gupta S, Avasthi A. Psychological correlates and psychiatric morbidity in patients with Dhat syndrome. Indian J Psychiatry. 2015;57(3):255–61. https://doi.org/10.4103/0019-5545.166637.

Grover S, Gupta S, Avasthi A. A follow-up study of patients with Dhat syndrome: treatment pattern, outcome, and reasons for dropout from treatment. Indian J Psychiatry. 2016c;58(1):49–56. https://doi.org/10.4103/0019-5545.174373.

Grover S, Gupta S, Mahajan S, Avasthi A. Pathway of care among patients with Dhat syndrome attending a psychosexual clinic in tertiary care center in North India. Ind Psychiatry J. 2016b;25(1):72–7. https://doi.org/10.4103/0972-6748.196040.

Grover S, Kate N, Avasthi A, Rajpal N, Umamaheswari V. Females too suffer from Dhat syndrome: a case series and revisit of the concept. Indian J Psychiatry. 2014a;56(4):388–92. https://doi.org/10.4103/0019-5545.146537.

Hanson BM, Aston KI, Jenkins TG, Carrell DT, Hotaling JM. The impact of ejaculatory abstinence on semen analysis parameters: a systematic review. J Assist Reprod Genet. 2018;35(2):213–20. https://doi.org/10.1007/s10815-017-1086-0.

Herbenick D, Fu TC, Wasata R, Coleman E. Masturbation prevalence, frequency, reasons, and associations with partnered sex in the midst of the COVID-19 pandemic: findings from a U.S. nationally representative survey. Arch Sex Behav. 2023;52(3):1317–31. https://doi.org/10.1007/s10508-022-02505-2.

Kar SK, Arafat SMY, Menon V. A bibliometric analysis of Dhat syndrome. Psychiatr Int. 2021a;2(4):379–85. https://doi.org/10.3390/psychiatryint2040029.

Kar SK, Menon V, Arafat SMY, Singh A, Das A, Shankar A, Sharma P, Perera S. Dhat syndrome: systematic review of epidemiology, nosology, clinical features, and management strategies. Asian J Psychiatr. 2021b;65:102863. https://doi.org/10.1016/j.ajp.2021.102863.

Kar SK, Sarkar S. Dhat syndrome: evolution of concept, current understanding, and need of an integrated approach. J Hum Reprod Sci. 2015;8(3):130–4. https://doi.org/10.4103/0974-1208.165143.

Kar SK, Singh A. Person centered management approach for the Dhat syndrome. Int J Pers Cent Med. 2016;6:4. https://doi.org/10.5750/ijpcm.v6i4.615.

Kar SK, Singh A. Where lies the fault in diagnosing Dhat syndrome among females? Understanding through a case study. Indian J Psychol Med. 2017;39(4):506–8. https://doi.org/10.4103/0253-7176.211742.

Khan N. *Dhat* syndrome in relation to demographic characteristics. Indian J Psychiatry. 2005;47(1):54–7. https://doi.org/10.4103/0019-5545.46077.

Lehman DR, Chiu CY, Schaller M. Psychology and culture. Annu Rev Psychol. 2004;55:689–714. https://doi.org/10.1146/annurev.psych.55.090902.141927.

Malhotra HK, Wig N. Dhat syndrome: a culture-bound sex neurosis of the orient. Arch Sex Behav. 1975;4(5):519–28. https://doi.org/10.1007/bf01542130.

Maruf MM, Khan MZR, Jahan N, Ahmed AU, Sadiq MS, Ferdush R. Sociodemographic profile and co-morbid symptoms among individuals with semen loss. Bangladesh J Med. 2021;33(1):64–9. https://doi.org/10.3329/bjm.v33i1.56792.

Mascherek A, Reidick MC, Gallinat J, Kühn S. Is ejaculation frequency in men related to general and mental health? Looking back and looking forward. Front Psychol. 2021;12:693121. https://doi.org/10.3389/fpsyg.2021.693121.

Mawhinney M, Mariotti A. Physiology, pathology and pharmacology of the male reproductive system. Periodontol. 2013;61(1):232–51. https://doi.org/10.1111/j.1600-0757.2011.00408.x.

Miah MAA, Al-Mamun MA, Khan S, Mozumder MK. Sexual myths and behavior of male patients with psychosexual dysfunction in sexual myths and behavior of male patients with psychosexual dysfunction in Bangladesh. Dhaka Univ J Psychol. 2015;39:89–100.

Mumford DB. The 'Dhat syndrome': a culturally determined symptom of depression? Acta Psychiatr Scand. 1996;94(3):163–7. https://doi.org/10.1111/j.1600-0447.1996.tb09842.x.

Nag M. Sexual behaviour and AIDS in India. Delhi: Vikas Publishing House; 1996.

Patel V, Pednekar S, Weiss H, Rodrigues M, Barros P, Nayak B, Tanksale V, West B, Nevrekar P, Kirkwood BR, Mabey D. Why do women complain of vaginal discharge? A population survey of infectious and pyschosocial risk factors in a south Asian community. Int J Epidemiol. 2005;34(4):853–62. https://doi.org/10.1093/ije/dyi072.

Prakash O. Lessons for postgraduate trainees about Dhat syndrome. Indian J Psychiatry. 2007;49(3):208–10. https://doi.org/10.4103/0019-5545.37324.

Prakash O, Kar SK. Dhat syndrome: a review and update. J Psychosexual Health. 2019;1(3–4):241–5. https://doi.org/10.1177/2631831819894769.

Prakash O, Kar SK, Rao TSS. Indian story on semen loss and related Dhat syndrome. Indian J Psychiatry. 2014;56(4):377–82. https://doi.org/10.4103/0019-5545.146532.

Prakash O, Meena K. Association between Dhat and loss of energy—a possible psychopathology and psychotherapy. Med Hypotheses. 2008;70(4):898–9. https://doi.org/10.1016/j.mehy.2007.09.010.

Rao TSS. History and mystery of Dhat syndrome: a critical look at the current understanding and future directions. Indian J Psychiatry. 2021;63(4):317–25. https://doi.org/10.4103/psychiatry.IndianJPsychiatry_791_20.

Saha M, Ray S, Goswami M, Kundu S, Saha P, Saha A, Maitra S, Talukdar A. An occult filarial infection presenting as chyluria with proteinuria: a case report and review of literature. BMJ Case Reports. 2012;2012:bcr0120125635. https://doi.org/10.1136/bcr.01.2012.5635.

Singh A, Tripathi A, Gupta B, Agarwal V. Pathways to care for Dhat (semen loss anxiety) syndrome: a study from North India. Int J Ment Health. 2016;45(4):253–61. https://doi.org/10.1080/00207411.2016.1238741.

Singh G. Dhat syndrome revisited. Indian J Psychiatry. 1985;27(2):119–22.

Strong YN, Li A, White ME, Razzak AN, Anderson DJ, Kaye AD, Herron EW, Khater NP, Bradley EC, Urits I. Dhat syndrome: epidemiology, risk factors, comorbidities, diagnosis, treatment, and management. Health Psychol Res. 2022;10(4):38759. https://doi.org/10.52965/001c.38759.

Sumathipala A, Siribaddana SH, Bhugra D. Culture-bound syndromes: the story of dhat syndrome. Br J Psychiatry. 2004;184:200–9. https://doi.org/10.1192/bjp.184.3.200.

Thakar VJ. Historical development of basic concepts of Ayurveda from Veda up to Samhita. Ayu. 2010;31(4):400–2. https://doi.org/10.4103/0974-8520.82024.

Udina M, Foulon H, Valdés M, Bhattacharyya S, Martín-Santos R. Dhat syndrome: a systematic review. Psychosomatics. 2013;54(3):212–8. https://doi.org/10.1016/j.psym.2012.09.003.

Verma RK, Sharma S, Singh R, Rangaiyan G, Pelto PJ. Beliefs concerning sexual health problems and treatment seeking among men in an Indian slum community. Cult Health Sex. 2003;5(3):265–76. https://doi.org/10.1080/136910501106356.

Wen JK, Wang CL. Shen-k'uei syndrome: a culture-specific sexual neurosis in Taiwan. Normal and abnormal behavior in Chinese culture, 1981; 357–369.

Whorton J. The solitary vice: the superstition that masturbation could cause mental illness. West J Med. 2001;175(1):66–8. https://doi.org/10.1136/ewjm.175.1.66.

Wig NN. Problems of mental health in India. J Clin Soc Psychiatry. 1960;17:48–53.

World Health Organization (WHO). WHO laboratory manual for the examination and processing of human semen. 5th ed. Geneva: World Health Organization; 2010.

GPSR Compliance

*The European Union's (EU) General Product Safety Regulation (GPSR) is a set of rules that requires consumer products to be safe and our obligations to ensure this.*

*If you have any concerns about our products, you can contact us on ProductSafety@springernature.com*

In case Publisher is established outside the EU, the EU authorized representative is:

Springer Nature Customer Service Center GmbH
Europaplatz 3
69115 Heidelberg, Germany

**Batch number: 09336648**

Printed by Printforce, the Netherlands